PRAISE FOR SOUKYA

'I hope that holistic health would make a valuable contribution to the future of humanity as the aim of holistic health is to achieve a happier and healthier living in a healthy environment.'

His Holiness The Dalai Lama

'What a wonderful experience! We go away rejuvenated and feeling a great deal better than when we came. Thank you for the warm welcome and friendly hospitality. Wonderful place of serenity and healing, with friendly, caring people.'

Archbishop Desmond Tutu and Leah Tutu

'I am in Bangalore to find out more about the International Holistic Health Centre, a spiritual quest to explore what it has to offer to a person's body and soul, to learn about the different traditional systems of medicine it has to offer and the different ways of helping a person to wholeness and harmony of body.'

Sarah, Duchess of York

'Dr Mathai's ayurvedic and medical centre, SOUKYA, in Bangalore is an extraordinary place for nurturing and healing. India should be proud to have a world-class facility that offers the best integrated approach to well-being. Dr Mathai is one of the most competent and brilliant holistic doctors in our world today.'

Dr Deepak Chopra

'SOUKYA has a tranquil and soothing ambience made exquisite by the smiling staff in housekeeping or the kitchen. The doctors at the treatment centre are both very knowledgeable and well informed, and the masseurs are fabulous—always smiling and dedicated. Dr and Mrs Mathai have created and continue to maintain this oasis of peace and good health. Many congratulations to Dr and Mrs Mathai for this truly excellent institution and the days of care and pampering I received here!'

Jayanthi Natarajan, Union Minister of State (Environment and Forests)

'Our ancient scriptures clearly reflect the awareness that the human being is an integrated entity and that any such successful treatment must involve the body, the mind, the emotions, and the deeper riches of the human spirit. This is the essence of holistic health which needs to be extensively propagated around the world.'

Dr Karan Singh, Former Federal Minister of Health (Government of India)

'SOUKYA is an oasis set in idyllic surroundings. It is the vision and far-sightedness of Dr and Mrs Mathai that have created this wonderland. Not only is the ambience perfect, but the maintenance is immaculate. I came here as a cynic but go back converted—this has been a holistic experience!! I came here sick in body and mind and go back convinced that I am on the road to a full recovery. The place, the doctors, and the entire staff have contributed to this wholesome experience. My wife joins me in sincerely thanking Dr and Mrs Mathai and everyone else. May God bless you.'

Mrs and Mr Gurbachan Jagat (Ex-Governor of Manipur)

DR MATHAI'S HOLISTIC HEALTH

Guide for Women

DR MATHAI'S HOLISTIC HEALTH
Guide for Women

Dr Issac Mathai

RANDOM HOUSE INDIA

Published by Random House India in 2013
1

Random House Publishers India Private Limited
Windsor IT Park, 7th Floor
Tower-B, A-1, Sector-125
Noida 201301, UP

Random House Group Limited
20 Vauxhall Bridge Road
London SW1V 2SA
United Kingdom

978 81 8400 195 2

Typeset in Sabon by R. Ajith Kumar

Printed and bound in India by Replika Press Private Limited

For sale in the Indian Subcontinent only

To my mother Dr Annamma Mathai,
my wife Suja Issac,
and my daughter Anna Issac—
the three most important women in my life

Contents

PART III: LIFESTYLE CONDITIONS

Foreword

It is ironic that I should have heard of Dr Issac Mathai, a brilliant Indian holistic doctor, through an American friend in New York. 'He is marvellous,' she said. 'I try and see him every time he comes here. You must meet him.' Always deeply interested in holistic medicine and in well-being, I decided to seek him out in Bangalore.

The first buildings of SOUKYA were up when I checked in for two weeks in early 2002. The main reception building housed all the medical facilities and treatment rooms. A few cottages for guests were ready; but what was laid out showed the promise of what was to come.

I have had experiences in both holistic centres and spas before. They are either medically excellent but poor in comfort, and lacking totally in aesthetics, or sumptuous in the environment and poor in all but the most perfunctory healing. The first cures illness, the second coddles. SOUKYA, in its early years, held the promise of both in one. And in the decade since, it has more than lived up to that promise.

Dr Mathai is a gifted healer. His wife Suja a careful nutritionist, with the eye of an aesthete and the demands of a stickler for order and cleanliness. The staff too is equally well trained. And the greatest joy (and surprise as this is India) is that each year it gets better.

As a dancer and performer who uses her body constantly and uses it hard, nothing gives me a greater sense of renewal than to go to SOUKYA. Dr Mathai's advice is straightforward and his understanding of health intuitive. I come away rejuvenated with all the niggling ailments gone, ready to take on the world. And my visits are the highlights of my year—I wish I could go twice a year.

I am sure this book will be a boon to all those in search of genuine wellness—not just freedom from ailments, but that sense of well-being that makes one smile at the world every day.

Dr Mallika Sarabhai
(Dancer, Activist)

Introduction

I GREW UP IN WAYANAD, KERALA, WHERE AYURVEDA IS ubiquitous. My father was a church priest and a reformer while my mother was a homeopath who ran a humble clinic and had immense faith in the powers of natural healing. It didn't come as a big surprise then that from a very early age I understood the benefits of considering more than one method of treatment.

I had a dream from childhood to create a holistic centre that offered the best integrative services. As destiny would have it, the possibility of taking over my mother's profession led me to do a course in homeopathy in Kottayam (Kerala) and eventually join my mother's clinic. It was while studying homeopathy in college that I took to meditation and also got myself enrolled in yoga classes. I saw how the recovery rate of the patients was better if one combined yoga with homeopathy. That's when I realized the future of medicine was in a holistic approach.

Most of us grow up with the idea that our bodies consist of independent parts. In school, we learn of the digestive, respiratory, or skeletal systems in isolation. We also have different names for people who treat different problems of the body—the gastroenterologist, the pulmonologist, the orthopaedist, the dentist…the list is endless. When I moved to England, I worked at an integrated medical centre called The

101 Clinic. Patients there had access to everything—from a physician to a spiritual healer. It was there that I discovered that many ailments, especially those which are chronic (constantly recurring), are best treated by a multi-pronged approach. I found that an intelligent combination of healing techniques dramatically improved results. For example, while I was treating patients with asthma using homeopathy alone, the success rate was around 60 percent. When I combined that with yoga therapy, breathing techniques, and nose washing, the success rate went up to 85 percent. It was no accident. That first experience of combining homeopathy and yoga had me convinced about the power of holistic healing.

Today, in association with a leading local cancer facility, I am working to integrate naturopathy and homeopathy with the prevalent chemotherapy method. I am not looking to replace or discredit chemotherapy. Quite the opposite, in fact. I am simply looking at how to improve the percentages by adding another dimension to the treatment. And the results so far have been very promising.

THE HOLISTIC WAY

As the name suggests, the holistic approach looks at the entire human body instead of individual parts. There are five levels of being—physical, mental, vital, intellectual, and spiritual. Holism incorporates, in addition to localized symptoms, the effects of psychological, social, environmental, and even economic influences on a person's health. By stepping back and taking a wider look, it is possible not only to treat but also prevent future recurrences. This is part of the philosophy of holistic medicine.

Holistic medicine has received more than its fair share of criticism and is often unfairly associated with miracle cures and spontaneous healing when nothing could be further from the truth. In fact, treatments based on holism tend to take time because they rely on stimulating the body's natural defence mechanisms to fight diseases. Diseases progress slowly. So too will the body's defences. Through this book, we will come across many common problems faced by women today. The purpose of this book is not just to describe them, but to suggest effective solutions to them.

There are several systems of medicine around the world, including ayurveda, herbalism, and homeopathy. Allopathy, or 'western medicine', is one of them too. It is often portrayed as being on one side while all other systems, condescendingly clubbed together under the term 'alternative medicine', are on the other. No single system can cure every disease. If it could, then all the others would be unnecessary, wouldn't they? By creating a dialogue between the systems, it becomes more likely that a doctor will find a suitable treatment and minimize or even eliminate side-effects entirely. Thus, allopathy too is part of holistic medicine. This is an important point and one that is often misunderstood; at no stage does holistic healing renounce western medicine. We simply see it in its place—as one of many possible alternatives.

The job of a holistic doctor is not to treat symptoms, but to stimulate the body to fight the root cause of illness. A holistic doctor is a catalyst for good health. Holism is more of an attitude than a discipline. It is something that can be adopted by anyone, and just requires a shift in a person's mindset.

Take menstrual pain for instance. Over the years, I have dealt with many women complaining about pain during menstruation. It is a common problem with many variations in intensity, frequency, and duration. Depending on these factors, a woman could:

1. Ignore the pain and hope it goes away. This is easier said than done and, in isolation, does nothing to help.
2. Self-medicate: She goes to a pharmacy and picks up an

over-the-counter painkiller. This is the worst thing she could possibly do. Even doing nothing is a better option.
3. Meet a General Practitioner (GP) or a gynaecologist and get a prescription.

Since painkillers target a specific symptom (namely, pain), their effect is almost immediate. The person walks away with the impression that the problem has been cured when in reality it is a symptom that has been silenced. This is not a long-term solution. There will be side-effects and the problem will return. With a slight shift in the person's approach to her own health, her recourse could now be to go to a holistic doctor who would do one of two things. Either the doctor would advise her on a natural course of treatment which may not yield results immediately, but treat the root cause of the symptoms. This will significantly benefit her in the long run. In case of extreme pain and discomfort, the doctor may prescribe a painkiller for immediate relief, for long enough that the homeopathic or ayurvedic treatment be allowed to work.

The physical effects of psychological stress

The mental state of an individual is a major factor in her physical well-being. People and relationships are an important part of a person's environment. Psychological suppression is enough to cause a chronic condition. I have come across many cases where a recurring physical symptom cannot be diagnosed by just medical tests. It was not until we delved into the psyche of the person, and created a profile based on the major developments in her life over the preceding year, that we found a permanent solution.

A few years ago, I was approached by a woman who complained of incessant shoulder pain. The usual tests were conducted, but gave us no answers. After six months, there was no improvement. It is at this point that I decided to arrange a private talk session with her, and asked her not to bring her husband along. It was time to look at things from a holistic perspective.

My first impression was that the shoulder pain was an escape mechanism that she had unintentionally developed in order to avoid having to do things that she did not want to do. This is not to say that I believed that she was faking the pain. It simply meant that her body had realized that this was an effective way to deal with unpleasant situations.

After more probing, I gathered that this was not the case. It was something else—something quite bizarre. She had convinced herself that her husband's life was at risk. She had decided that his brother and sister-in-law were plotting to poison him and take over their business. The paranoia grew to a point where any mention of her husband's brother triggered a bout of shoulder pain.

With this new information, my course of action was clear. I referred her to a psychologist whose therapy included hypnosis. A few sessions later, her pain was gone. This is what the holistic approach teaches us. Once the root cause is established—be it psychological, physical, environmental—the treatment has to be aimed directly at the cause. The symptoms will naturally disappear as a result.

Symptoms Are the Last Stage in the Development of a Disease

Absence of symptoms is not a sure sign of good health. The appearance of symptoms of a disease is the last step in a gradual process of the malfunctioning of a system. Even something as trivial as a sneeze is the culmination of a thousand little processes within our bodies. That doesn't mean that we should all turn into hypochondriacs and live in fear. But it does mean that it is up to us to take care of our own bodies as a matter of habit, well before symptoms start to pop up.

THE DOCTOR IS AN ARCHITECT

Doctors should be health specialists, not disease specialists. Unfortunately, many people, including doctors themselves, lose sight of this. In order for a person to live healthy, it is imperative that they take control of their own lives, and allow doctors to guide them as necessary. This includes things like getting a second opinion from another doctor. This is especially important when a suggested course of action involves hormone therapy or risky surgery. As long as the condition is not so far gone as to require immediate emergency surgery, a second opinion is always recommended.

One simple and extremely effective tool in maintaining good health is finding a good local primary physician. Most of us have a tendency, at the slightest provocation, to run to a large hospital and seek treatment from the best specialist. In their capacity as an architect, a good physician can recommend alternative treatments before directing a person to a specialist. Developing a relationship with a physician allows them to understand your medical history better. For all their expertize, specialists who spend no more than five minutes with a patient before diagnosing them cannot compete with such physicians.

No single doctor can be an expert at every system of medicine. Indeed, each system has enough in it for more than a lifetime's worth of study. As a homeopath, my approach to holistic medicine is not to try to understand every aspect of allopathy, naturopathy, or ayurveda myself. It is to be able to recognize what these other systems have to offer, and then be in a position to recommend to a patient an expert in some other system, if necessary. If the best option is surgery, then so be it—as long as it is the best option, not the quickest or most convenient.

Soukya

Over the years, I have travelled around the world, immersing myself in local systems of medicine, from homeopathy to Chinese acupuncture. After seeing the success we had at The 101 Clinic with our multifaceted approach, it dawned on me that the perfect environment for holistic healing was not a large city, and certainly not one whose weather was as dismal as it was in England. India has the largest collection of indigenous, traditional forms of medicine. What better place to create a holistic health retreat? This was the rationale behind the development of SOUKYA, a completely holistic healing centre located on the outskirts of Bangalore.

Women's health

The female body is especially complex. As with any complex entity, it can be affected by myriad problems. It is critical to understand them and take precautions to avoid them.

A young woman in India today faces challenges unlike any in the past. Carrying forward the roles of homemaker and mother from previous generations, she also balances a full-time career. The pressure that a young woman is under to succeed from an early age can have a devastating effect on her body.

The notion of a nuclear family is relatively new to India. As a society, we have not yet figured out how to arrive at a suitable balance between a prosperous career and good health. I come across women all the time who tell me that they simply do not have the time to eat properly. Eating unhealthy, convenient food is the solution to the problem of shortage of time. This cycle begins in the later teenage years, when staying up all night to study is seen as normal or even necessary. This continues into one's professional life as well. Stimulated by financial incentives, it is easy to make the wrong choices for one's body. Often the repercussions of this do not show until it is too late. And a lot of the damage done is long-term and irreversible.

A woman's peak childbearing years can be dramatically affected by the subtle but incremental abuse sustained right from the early teen years. It is essential to keep this in mind from an early age. I have dealt with people who, at the age of 35, after years of irregular eating, sleeping, and attempts at quick-fix solutions to problems as they pop up, are desperate to get pregnant, but cannot. Twenty years of abuse cannot be undone in a year or two.

The secret to a successful career and family is in the ability to find the perfect balance. I wish there was a simple answer to the question of how to find that balance. If there is, I certainly have not found it.

Don't wait to repair your body only after it breaks down. Pay attention to what it is telling you. Use this book to restore your body's natural balance by treating the body as a whole—mind, body, and spirit. After all, good health is much more than the absence of a disease.

Why This Book?

There are a number of books concerned with illustrating problems associated with certain conditions. Not this one. My aim is to tackle problems head on with an eye on solutions which can be practised at every level—from simple home remedies to yoga and then further on.

Of course, the best way to deal with health problems is not to allow them to develop in the first place. Prevention is easier, less expensive, and more efficient than a cure. Through a combination of factors such as diet, exercise, meditation, and control of the environment, we will look at how best to reduce the risk of some common ailments, and also at different and effective therapies and methodologies.

The internet now allows people access to vast amounts of information. Unfortunately, not all of this information is accurate, and this can be dangerous. The source of information on women's health should be sound. Glossy magazines, which ostensibly speak of women's health, focus more often only on sex. With all of this information bombarding us all the time, it is important for women to find a trustworthy source. This is where my book is different.

The book is broadly divided into three sections, with the underlying approach to all of them being holism. The first part deals with common body conditions of both men and women, but the focus, however, will be on how they affect women. The second part looks at gynaecological conditions that affect women of all ages. And the final section deals with lifestyle conditions such as stress and ageing.

To quote British poet Robert Browning, 'Ignorance is not innocence, but sin.' It is up to each one of us to take matters into our own hands. And the first step in doing that is by understanding how our bodies work.

Part I

Common Body Conditions

THE AIM OF THE FIRST PART OF THIS BOOK IS TO EMPOWER you to make intelligent and informed decisions with regard to your body and health.

There are constant physiological and psychological changes that take place throughout the various stages of your life, and in order to understand the many challenges you may face as you go along, this book will serve as a constant companion.

For the sake of convenience, let us divide a woman's lifespan into:

- The teens to age 25
- The early married years to age 35
- The pre-menopausal woman
- Menopause and beyond
- Old age

In the teen years, there are several hormonal changes that take place and sometimes a young woman has problems, for example, with her menstrual cycle, or an over/underactive thyroid.

Around the time that you marry, have children, and take on the many responsibilities of a home and family, all the while balancing those with a career, there are various facets of your life that vie for priority. Your children, husband, career, extra-curricular interests, friends, family, and everything but your health has your attention. With the dissolution of the 'joint family' and with the increasing dependence on the wife/mother to balance the household, there is an untold amount of stress on today's 30-something woman. For various reasons, you just don't pay enough attention to yourself and forget about the well-being of your body; so all this plus a lack of exercise puts stress on you that can spark off ill-health in this stage of life.

As you read on about the common body conditions that confront a majority of women today, I urge you to keep a few things in mind. The modern, urban working woman is beset with more challenges than her predecessors or even her rural counterparts ever encountered. Given the balancing acts you have to perform, your various responsibilities both at work and at home, and the resulting stress and unhealthy lifestyle, there is a higher predisposition to health-related problems. It is important to recognize this and understand that there is much you can do on your journey through life to preempt and prepare for these battles, using strategies provided in this book.

CHAPTER ONE

Musculoskeletal System

WHETHER IT'S DUE TO A FALL FROM A STAIRCASE OR TOO much physical workout, activities of everyday life can sometimes bring on muscle pain and related body aches. The musculoskeletal system is the largest and one of the most important systems in the human body for it is what keeps us upright and facilitates movement. Made up of bones, tendons, ligaments, cartilage, muscles, and joints, it allows us to move and provides form, support, and stability to the body. The musculoskeletal system's primary functions include supporting the body, allowing motion, and protecting vital organs. There are, however, diseases and disorders that may adversely affect the function and overall effectiveness of the system.

Osteoporosis

Have you ever broken an arm or a leg at a young age and thought to yourself, *How could this happen to me? I'm not 80 yet!*

I often find myself repeating the same thing to my patients that osteoporosis can happen to anyone at any age, though it is often considered to be a condition that frail elderly women develop. However, the damage from osteoporosis begins much earlier in life. Because peak bone density is reached at approximately 25 years of age, it is important to build strong bones by then, so that the bones remain strong later in life. Adequate calcium intake is an essential part of building strong bones. Osteoporosis presents itself with symptoms like joint pains, difficulty in standing, difficulty sitting up straight, and the 'stooping' position often seen among elderly people.

Simply put, osteoporosis is a disease of the bones that leads to an increased risk of fracture. It literally means porous bones and implies the thinning of bone tissue and loss of bone density over time. It is a condition caused by a reduction in the quality of the bones, which leads to weakness of the skeleton and an increased risk of fractures. Due to a low bone mineral density (BMD), the bone becomes compressible, like a sponge, and therefore fragile.

It is estimated that 1 in every 3 women over the age of 50 suffers from fractures due to osteoporosis.

Why does osteoporosis occur?

Osteoporosis occurs when there is an imbalance between new bone formation and old bone reabsorption. As we age, there are many factors that cause the bones to demineralize and these make the bones brittle. The early stage of demineralization is called osteopenia and, if undetected and untreated, leads to osteoporosis.

Causes

The following factors lead to an increased risk of osteoporosis:

- Female gender.
- Asian race.
- Family history of osteoporosis.

- Cigarette smoking.
- Excessive alcohol consumption.
- History of fractures as an adult.
- Lack of exercise.
- Poor nutrition and poor general health.
- Malabsorption of minerals.
- Low estrogen levels in women.
- Chemotherapy.
- Immobility due to prolonged illness or surgery.
- Hyperparathyroidism: Parathyroid hormones maintain blood calcium levels by removing calcium from the bone. In the case of hyperparathyroidism, excessive production of parathyroid hormones causes too much calcium removal from the bones, leading to osteoporosis.
- Vitamin D deficiency: This leads to inadequate absorption of calcium from diet.
- Long-term use of medicines like heparin, anti-seizure medicines, and corticosteroids.

Common symptoms

Osteoporosis itself has no specific symptoms; its main consequence is the increased risk of bone fractures. It can be present without any symptoms for decades until the bone breaks. Therefore, people may not be aware of their osteoporosis until they suffer a painful fracture. The symptom associated with osteoporotic fractures usually is pain; the location of the pain depends on the location of the fracture. Over the years, repeated spinal fractures can lead to chronic lower back pain as well as loss of height and/or curving of the spine due to collapse of the vertebrae. This collapse gives individuals a hunched-back appearance.

Hip fractures typically occur as a result of a fall. With osteoporosis, hip fractures can occur as a result of trivial accidents. Also, these fractures may heal slowly or poorly after surgical repair because of poor healing of the bone.

Types

Primary Type I or postmenopausal osteoporosis is common in women who have reached menopause.

Primary Type II or senile osteoporosis can occur in both men and women usually after the age of 75.

Secondary osteoporosis can occur in both men and women at any age, and usually occurs due to predisposing medical problems or prolonged use of medications like steroids.

Prevention

- Use of calcium: Osteoporosis is a condition affecting bones due to reduced calcium, making them porous and easily breakable. This happens as a result of decreased calcium absorption, reduced level of estrogen in women post-menopause leading to reduced calcium absorption, decreased Vit-D, lack of weight-bearing exercises, and as an after-effect of certain steroids. With regular intake of adequate amount of calcium, especially in women during the fertile age, this condition could be largely prevented. Adequate intake of calcium in a day is useful in preventing osteoporosis. Food sources of calcium include low-fat dairy products such as milk, yogurt, cheese, and ice cream; dark green, leafy vegetables such as broccoli, collard greens, bok choy, and spinach; sardines and salmon with bones; tofu; almonds; sesame seeds, green gram, quinoa; and foods fortified with calcium, such as orange juice, cereals, and breads. The sources of phytoestrogens are soya and its products, flaxseeds, yam, colocasia, alfalfa, fennel etc.
- Ragi could be taken as porridge, in idli, dosa, roti etc. This can also be included in the flour for phulkas/chapatis.
- Vitamin D: Vitamin D plays an important role in calcium absorption and bone health. Food sources of Vitamin D

include egg yolks, saltwater fish, and cod liver.

- Exercise: Like muscle, bone is living tissue that responds to exercise by becoming stronger. Exercises like walking, hiking, jogging, climbing stairs, weight training, tennis, and dancing are helpful in prevention of osteoporosis.

Holistic approach

Homeopathic and ayurvedic internal medications help set right hormonal imbalance, if any, improve calcium absorption, and supplement necessary calcium.

Homeopathy

Homeopathic medicines in their biochemic form (tissue salts which help in combating the insufficiency of organic salts in the tissues and cells of the body) help as supportive treatments in building the strength of the bones and in preventing further damage to the skeletal system. There are 12 biochemic remedies. These medicines help in absorption of the calcium from regular diet. Homeopathic medicines such as Phosphorous, Calcarea phos, Silica, Merc sol act in a supportive, preventive, and stabilizing role to enable the reabsorption of calcium from external source.

Naturopathy

Naturopathic treatments mainly aim at improving the body's metabolism, thereby improving calcium absorption. Acupuncture can definitely relieve back pain by relieving the stiffness/spasming of muscles. Localized as well as distal points are used. Depending on the condition, acupuncture is done with or without stimulation. Massage with medicated oils and medicated pouches too relieve stiffness of the muscles and reduce inflammation, if any. Hydrotherapy like spinal bath, immersion bath, and the jets also help.

Ayurveda

Ayurvedic treatments like Navarakizhi, Nasya, and Vasti too help in improving the bone density and setting right metabolism.

Yoga

Specific yogic postures like Bhujangasana, Dhanurasana, Trikonasana, Vrikshasana, Garudasana, Gomukhasana, Baradwajasana, Sarvangasana, Sethubandhasana, Salabhasana, Ardha Matsyendrasana etc. help improve bone density. Along with this, deep breathing, sectional breathing, Nadi Shodhana, Ujjayi Pranayama help as well.

JOINT PAIN

Joint ache is a condition which is characterized by pain and sometimes stiffness of a joint. This is sometimes associated with swelling as well.

Take the case of Hitesh, a senior business analyst at a multinational company in Gurgaon, who has regular bouts of joint pain and stiffness in his body. When he came to me for treatment, he told me that his pain had become increasingly worse over time and he feared getting crippled for life.

Pain in the joints can be caused due to overexertion, injuries, arthritis, muscle pain, bursitis etc. There can sometimes be swelling and redness of the joint if the inflammation is very severe.

Causes

The causes of joint pain can be broadly categorized under:

- Wear and tear.
- Injuries.

- Weight.
- Lack of exercise.
- Muscle loss.
- Stress.
- Inflammation of the joints.
- Metabolic disorders.
- Bone diseases.
- Tumours or cancer.

Prevention

- Fruits and vegetables cut the risk of arthritis and reduce inflammation. Maintaining overall good health is important to have healthy joints. Exercising regularly to maintain ideal weight helps in reducing joint degeneration. However, you must keep in mind not to overdo the exercises.
- Control weight: Minimizing weight can reduce forces directed to weight-bearing joints.
- Eat a healthy diet: Antioxidants have an anti-inflammatory effect on the body. Deep coloured fruits and vegetables are our best source of antioxidants. Thus it is important to eat a diet rich with these foods. As oxidative stress is reduced, so is inflammation in the body.
- Protect joints: Muscles are not the only means of protecting joints from abnormal stress. For weight-bearing joints such as feet, ankles, knees, and hips, wearing the right shoes can be invaluable.

Holistic approach

Holistic approach always helps in strengthening the joints and tendons and slows down degeneration of the joints. As per the holistic approach, we try to analyse the symptoms at a very early stage by understanding the patient's history and physical examinations. The treatments involve those that can improve the secretion of synovial fluid so as to improve lubrication of the joints and enable smooth, painless movements. Simultaneously, treatments to strengthen the surrounding muscles, ligaments, and tendons and to cure any inflammatory changes are done. This ensures control of the degenerative process. Internal medications too help with the process.

Homeopathy

Homeopathic medicines like Rhus Tox, Bryonia, Cal phos, Ruta, Arnica etc. help in treating joint pains.

Naturopathy

Naturopathic treatments like Infra-red, acupuncture, mud packs, hot mud applications, and compresses are few treatments which are beneficial in arthritis and joint complaints.

Ayurveda

Treatments like Abhyanga, Choorna Swedam, Lepam, Pichu, PPS, Nasyam, Vasti, Padabhyanga, and Kativasti, when combined with good bed rest, can yield positive results.

The treatments vary according to the condition. In suitable conditions, treatments like upanaha swedam, special herbal applications, pelvic traction help.

According to ayurveda, joint pain is because of degenerative changes. So the basic principle is to slow down the degenerative process and slowly reverse the changes. Degenerative changes occur due to wear and tear.Ageing and inappropriate postures, movements and habits bring on this process. This could affect any organ or system in the body, but it harms mainly the joints. The synovial fluid secretion reduces as a result, causing gritty movements. This leads to tissue damage, be it the bone, muscles, ligaments, or tendons. This causes painful joints and joint movements.

External applications like lepam and pichu are done for this purpose and Choorna Swedam, PPS, Navara, and Pizhichil help to nourish the body and improve the organ functions. They also remove sluggishness.

Herbs like Guduchi, Bala, Guggulu, Eranda, Nirgundi, and Rasna are all helpful.

Yoga

Stretching and relaxation helps to release the muscle stiffness and also lubricates the joints.

Simple yogic exercises with breathing (Sukshma Vyayama), Suryanamaskars, and postures specific to the involved joints should be practiced.

Back Pain

Back pain is pain felt in the back, which usually originates from the muscles, nerves, bones, joints, or other structures in the spine.

Shilpi Sakhuja, a 34-year-old graphic designer, would be under so much pressure to meet the given deadlines that she would be sitting in front of her Mac Notebook for eight hours at a stretch! Over the years, I have seen so many women like Shilpi who come to me complaining of back pain. Sitting in the same position for so many hours wreaks havoc on your body, and may thus manifest itself at times in the form of back pain.

Causes

Back pain (backache) is the most common disability in persons less than 45 years of age. The incidence of lower backache is greater among women.

Muscle, nerve, ligament stress, fibroid tumour, menstrual cramps, pregnancy, endometriosis etc. are some of the female issues that could lead to back pain. Backaches during pregnancy are very common. Around 80 percent of women will experience back pain at some point during their pregnancies. The severity of this pain can range from mild discomfort after standing for long periods of time to debilitating pain that interferes with their daily lives.

Backaches can be an outcome of different illnesses. The pain may occur in combination with other symptoms depending on the underlying issue. Back pains due to infection or inflammation may be accompanied by a fever. Back pain due to fibromyalgia (a long-term condition that causes pain all over the body) may include symptoms such as insomnia and fatigue.

Types of back pain

The pain can often be divided into neck pain, upper back pain, and lower back pain or tailbone pain. The pain may stay in one place or radiate to other areas like the arms and hands when the pain is felt in the upper back, or to the legs and feet when it is felt in the lower back. Pain may include weakness, numbness, or tingling.

Prevention

The important tips for the prevention of backache include:

- Taking steps to reduce weight, if obese. Being overweight increases the chances of having a backache considerably.
- Muscles should be well-conditioned by maintaining standing and sitting postures.
- Maintaining the same postures for a long period of time is hazardous.
- Avoid lifting heavy weights. If lifting is required, never bend at the waist or stoop to pick up the object. Instead, lower the body to the level of the object by bending the knees. Grasp the object, hold it close to the body, and raise yourself with your legs, all the while keeping your back straight.
- Sleep on a firm mattress.

- Wear low-heeled shoes.
- Eat a healthy and balanced diet which is rich in fibre. Food adequate in calcium and Vit-D have to be included.
- Sex should be avoided during acute phase of pain as it can aggravate the same.
- Stress and strain increases the chances of backache, so relaxation is very important. Yoga and meditation are beneficial tools for relaxation.
- Regular exercises will strengthen the muscles and hence have a pivotal role in prevention of backache.

Holistic approach

Homeopathy

The approach in homeopathy comprises of a holistic view of the case. In acute pain, homeopathic remedies will relieve the backache. If the problem is persistent or recurring, a constitutional medicine is given based on the holistic view of the case. Medicines like Rhus Tox, Bryonia, Kali Carb, Arnica, Hypericum, Ruta, Symphytum, Mag Phos, Bellis Per are helpful.

Naturopathy

Acupuncture: Stimulation with fine needles to specific energy points on the back helps in relieving immediate pain, stiffness, and spasms. If the condition is severe, electro acupuncture is recommended.

Hydrotherapy: Treatments like spinal baths, hip baths, douches/jet therapy, and vichy showers help relax the back muscles.

Mud therapy: Hot mud is used on the back to relieve muscle spasms.
Acupressure: Stimulating the specific points on the back helps in relieving lower back pain and stiffness.

Ayurveda

Ayurvedic treatments like Katibasti, Abhyanga, Patra Potala Swedam, Marmalepam, Vasti, and Nasyam help to relieve the stiffness of the back, prevent degeneration of bones, strengthen the muscles and thus reduce the pain. Internal medications are also prescribed to alleviate pain.

Yoga

This will help to strengthen the back muscles. Practice backward bending exercises/postures. Along with this you can do specific breathing exercises. These exercises improve blood circulation to the back muscles and maintain the normal space between any two vertebrae.

Specific yogic postures like Bhujangasana, Salabhasana, Sethubandhasana, Pawanmuktasana, Makarabhyasa, Naukasana, Katichakrasana, Parswa Chakrasana are all helpful.

Diet

Diet plays a key role in the holistic approach for the treatment of backache. Back pain can be reduced by providing proper nutrition to the body. Eat a diet rich in calcium and protein. Include fresh fruits and vegetables, whole-grain cereals, and wholewheat breads in your diet. Limit the intake of soft drinks, candy bars, ice cream, cookies, and other sweets, because they tend to increase the weight and cause strain on the back.

Slipped Disc

Slipped disc, also called 'spinal disc herniation', is a condition affecting the spine in which a tear in the outer, fibrous ring of an inter-vertebral disc allows the soft, central portion to bulge out and cause nerve root compression.

I get many cases of slipped disc where patients don't even realize the severity of their condition. They come complaining of an ache in the neck ranging from mild to acute pain. It is only when the pain extends to other parts of the body that such patients realize the severity of the condition. What they had previously dismissed as a sign of stress and ageing is actually a more serious condition that needs treatment. In most of these cases, the cause of the problem turns out to be a herniated disc in the cervical vertebrae which presses on the spinal nerve, thus causing pain.

Causes

Factors that lead to a slipped disc include ageing with associated degeneration, loss of elasticity of the discs and supporting structures, injury from improper lifting (especially if accompanied by twisting or turning), and excessive strain forces associated with physical activities.

Common symptoms

Symptoms of a herniated disc can vary depending on the location of the herniation and the types of soft tissue that become involved. They can range from little or no pain—if the disc is the only tissue injured—to severe and unrelenting neck or low back pain that will radiate into the regions served by affected nerve roots that are irritated or impinged by the herniated material.

Prevention

Prevention of slipped disc can be achieved by taking care of the following:

❖ Exercise: Core-muscle strengthening helps stabilize and support the spine. Check with your doctor before resuming high-impact activities such as jogging or tennis. Regular exercise can improve the overall strength and tone of the supporting muscles and structures. Low back exercises are particularly important to prevent recurrent back injury.

- Maintain good posture: Good posture reduces the pressure on spine and discs. Keep your back straight and aligned, particularly when sitting for long periods. Lift heavy objects properly, making the legs and not the back do most of the work. Use proper techniques while performing strenuous exercise. The worst possible combination of activities for spine is heavy lifting while bending and twisting simultaneously.
- Maintain a healthy weight: Excess weight puts more pressure on the spine and discs, making them more susceptible to herniation.
- Use of a spine brace during heavy lifting is advised. Its use is to keep back straight and encourage proper lifting technique.

Holistic approach

Back pain being a very common disease in women, can be tacked very well with a holistic approach. Though this is a purely physical condition, treating it holistically gives better and longlasting results. Through the evaluation, we try to assess the patient's posture and habits. Treatments to correct the damage to the tissues and to enable the repositioning of the disc are done. This is followed by treatments to strengthen the muscles and the tissues. Simple changes in posture, reassessing your habits, and right movements help.

Homeopathy

Internal homeopathic medicines like Ruta, Hypericum, Arnica, Rhus Tox etc. help in relieving the pain. Constitutional homeopathic medicines help in addressing the problem from the root cause.

Naturopathy

Naturopathic treatments like wax therapy, hot mud packs, hydrotherapy fomentation, Infra-red light treatments, pelvic packs, spinal baths, and acupuncture help along with other treatments.

Ayurveda

The strength of ayurveda in the area of spinal ailments is globally appreciated. Since it addresses the root cause of the issue, the results are better than surgical procedures. Ayurveda holds that the herniated disc is a result of vitiation of the three principal 'doshas', especially the Vata. Treatment in ayurveda is aimed at restoring the equilibrium through correction of the underlying functional in-equilibrium. The treatment comprises of Elimination (Sodhanam) of the accumulated toxic products and metabolism of the disease process, Pacification (Samanam) and correction of the entities responsible for altered functioning, and Rasayanam (Rejuvenation) of the bodily tissue, to regain and maintain natural strength and vitality.

Therapies like Abhyanga, Nasyam, Patra Potala Swedam, Choorna Swedam, Pizhichil, Shirodhara, Kadeevasthi, Greevavasthi, Navarakizhi, and Vasti are done as per the need and condition of the patient. These therapies are directed towards relieving the inflammatory changes and herniation, releasing the spasms and nerve compressions in the affected area, strengthening the supportive tissues holding the spine/joints, nourishing the entire spine, and rehydrating the discs. Usually the treatment period varies between 3–5 weeks according to the severity of the illness.

In 4–6 weeks, a majority of the patients find their symptoms are relieved without surgery. If a patient can come for the treatment in early stages, even total cure without recurrence is possible. Internal ayurvedic medicines are also necessary.

Yoga

Specific asanas like the Bhujangasana, Ardha Chakrasana, Ushtrasana, Sethubandhasana, Kriyas, breathing and relaxation techniques, and meditation help in curing back pain.

Diet

Avoid gassy food items which can increase pain.

Minor cases can be handled at home in consultation with the doctor. Treatment at home includes application of hot or cold packs and basic pain relievers. As the condition improves, specific neck/back stretching/strengthening exercises can be done.

Bed rest or limited activity for several days followed by gradual increase in activity over the next few weeks is advised. People with back pain have been shown to recover more quickly with normal activity as long as lifting, bending, and straining is limited.

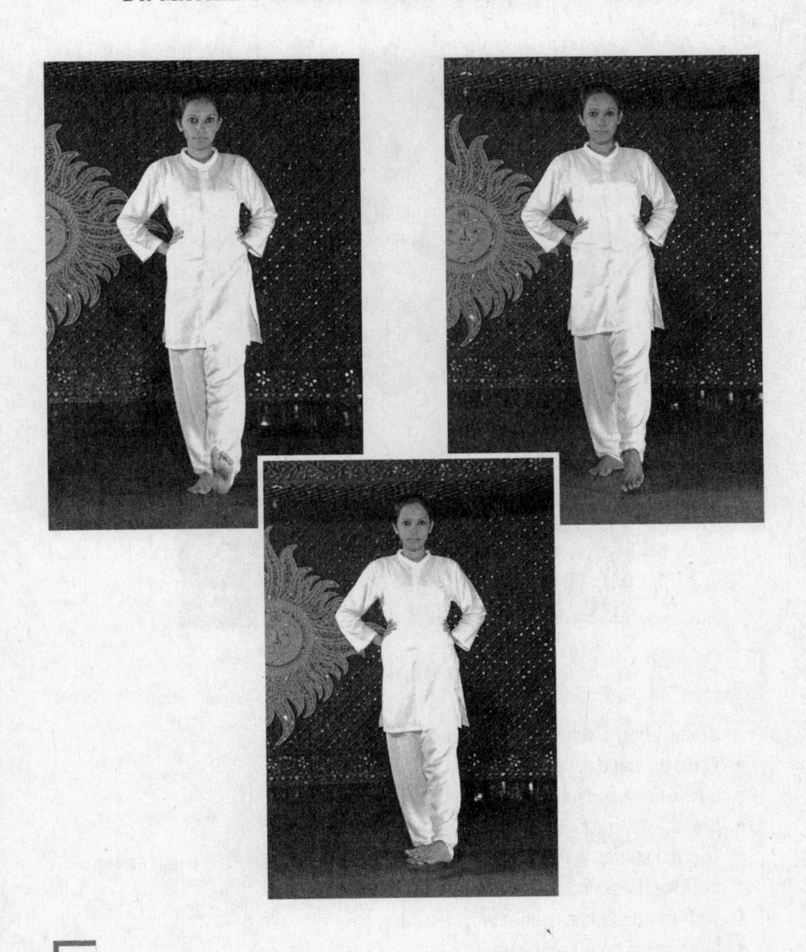

Ankle Movements

- Lift the ankle upwards as you inhale, exhale and bend it down.
- Slowly move the ankle sideways.
- Slowly and gently rotate the ankle. Repeat it in the opposite direction.

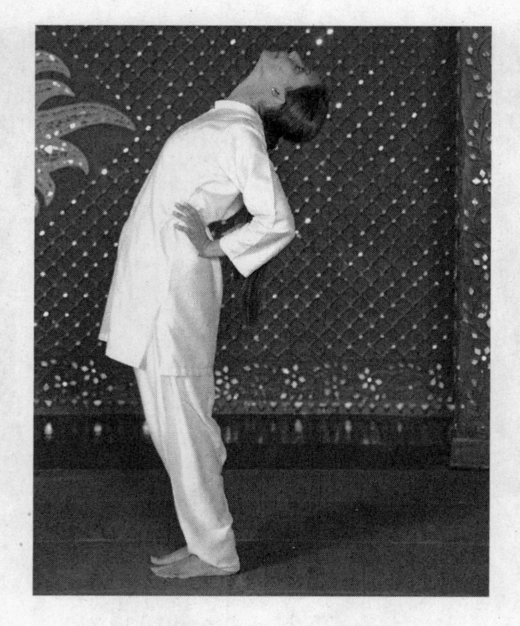

Ardha Chakrasana

- Stand straight with the legs together.
- Place the hands on the respective hip.
- Inhale and bend backwards from the waist.
- Breathe normally while you hold the posture.
- Feel the stretch in the shoulders, chest, and abdomen. Feel the compression in the lower back and spine.
- With an exhalation, gently straighten the spine.
- Release the hands and relax.

Benefits

- This posture relieves back pain
- It aligns spinal vertebra

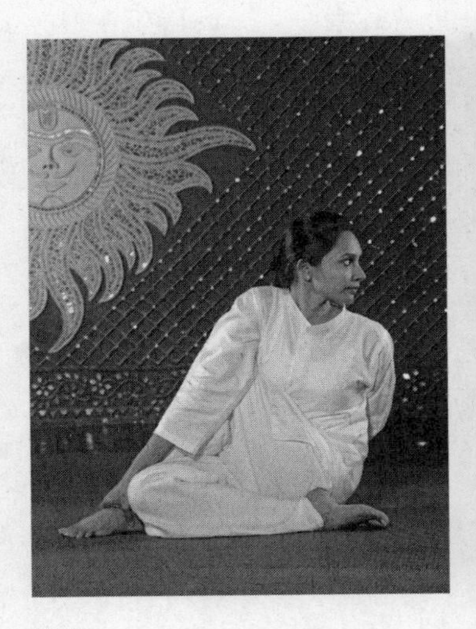

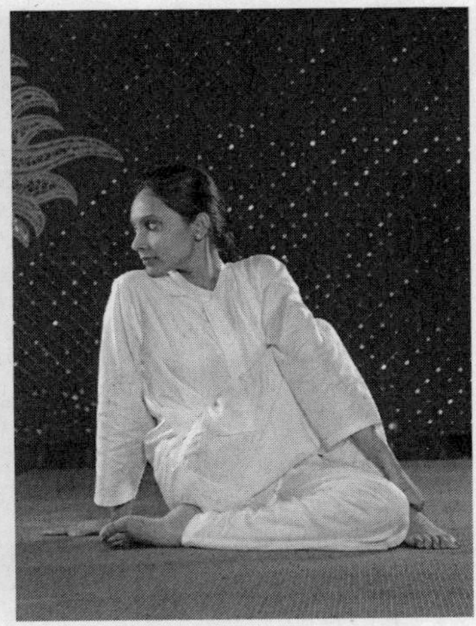

Ardha Matsyendrasana

- Sit with the legs stretched.
- Take the right leg from below the left leg, right foot by the side of left hip.
- Cross the left leg and place the left foot by the outer side of right knee.
- Turn the body to the left with an inhalation and hold the left ankle with the right hand.
- Cross the left hand across the spine.
- Exhale and turn the head to look to the back.
- Hold the posture with normal breathing.
- Feel the compression in the abdomen, stretch in the neck, shoulders, and hips.
- With inhalation, turn the head forward.
- As you exhale, release the right hand, then release the left; turn the torso forward and straighten the right knee.
- Relax and practice it on the other side.

Benefits

This is the asana which helps in controlling diabetes • Its practice relieves constipation and bloatedness; improves digestion • It relieves stiffness from the whole body

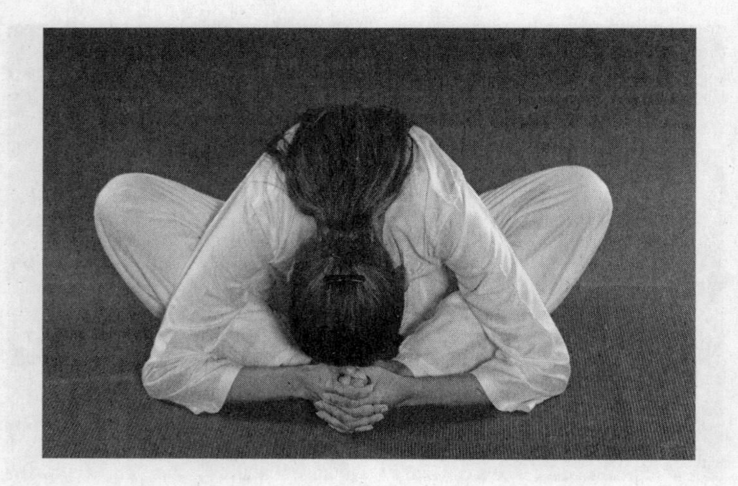

Baddha Konasana

- Sit with the back straight.
- Bend the legs at the knees and join the soles of the feet.
- Try to keep the knees completely on the ground.
- Hold the toes or ankles with your hands.
- Now take a deep inhalation.
- As you exhale bend forward and try to touch the forehead to the toes.
- Try not to raise the knees.
- Do not overstretch.
- Try to hold it where ever you can comfortably.
- Breathe normally.
- With every exhalation, try and bend down further.
- As you inhale, slowly straighten the spine, release the hands, and straighten the legs.
- Relax in sitting position.

Benefits

This asana strengthens the pelvic region, tones the thighs, and improves digestion • This is particularly beneficial in women of fertile age group

CHAPTER TWO

Digestive System

IT'S THE MIDDLE OF THE WEEK AND YOU ARE ATTENDING AN office meeting, trying your best to focus on the PowerPoint presentation on monthly sales figures. But the gurgling sound emanating from your stomach is making concentration increasingly difficult, not to mention, embarrassing, in a room full of peers and senior executives. Try as you may to shield the sound through your incessant coughing, their stares are enough to tell you that the technique is not working. So all you can do at that point is cough some more, and impatiently wait for the meeting to get over. An hour later, you rush to the bathroom to take care of the 'problem' that has been troubling you all morning. 'I am never eating that hot pepperoni pizza again', you tell yourself sitting on the toilet seat.

Pretty embarrassing, isn't it? But diarrhoea and other related digestive disorders are ones that most of us encounter on a daily basis. In fact, diarrhoea is the second most common cause of infant deaths worldwide!

It's a known fact that digestive system is one of the most important mechanisms in the body, but it is also one we tend to take for granted, choosing to focus more on our hair and skin. We all know that food cannot be absorbed in the body directly and needs to be broken down into smaller molecules for smooth digestion. The role of a well-functioning digestive system is that it allows us to break and digest food more easily, further processing food into nutrients and dispensing them through our blood stream.

Since the digestive system has the tendency to get upset easily, it is important that we take great care of it. But in today's day and age, an unhealthy lifestyle, irregular eating patterns, and physical and emotional stress are making this increasingly difficult. The result is that most of the times we tend to take digestive issues lightly in the hustle and bustle of our daily life. This, in turn, takes a toll on our health, which, if ignored in the long run, can have serious repercussions on the body.

The most common ailments associated with an unhealthy digestive system are indigestion, acidity, ulcers, constipation, anorexia/bulimia and gall stones. It is important that we have a correct understanding of all these in order to be able to manage them effectively.

Indigestion

Sumit Sachdeva is an IT professional with a big multinational company. Single and in his early 30s, he resides alone in his plush bachelor pad in Gurgaon where he hosts quite a few parties. He prides himself on being the perfect party host and is known for being quite a regular at all the happening events in town. But on most days after his revelry, he usually wakes up with a heavy stomach, complaining of bloating and heaviness in the abdomen, with occasional pain, especially in the upper part of the abdomen. This is often accompanied by belching, nausea, and heartburn.

When I met Sumit in my clinic, he talked to me about how his condition had increasingly become worse due to unhealthy eating habits. Having a sweet tooth, he gorged on mithais and laddus. Living alone was another excuse for him to skip meals, order takeaways, and eat at restaurants. Plus, a weak digestive system since childhood had made the situation worse. I confronted him and told him that his singlehood had become a crutch for him to justify wrong eating habits.

I advised him to eat small portions of food at regular intervals, to avoid heavy and oily food for some time, to drink about 2 litres of water every day, and prescribed to him a few homeopathic medicines. Gradually, his digestion came back on track.

But here I want to pause and tell you how no two people will have the same problem. And in that regard, the solutions to their problems will differ too. Early detection of any ailment is central to its cure. You must have heard of numerous cases where grave illnesses like cancer get cured because they were taken care of in the initial stages itself. The same applies for all ailments in general.

Causes

Indigestion can be attributed to many causes, some of which are given below:

- Indigestion can be caused by a condition in the digestive tract such as gastroesophageal reflux disease (GERD), peptic ulcer disease, cancer, or abnormality of the pancreas or bile ducts.
- Non-gastrointestinal diseases such as diabetes, thyroid disease, hyperthyroidism (overactive parathyroid glands), and severe kidney diseases.
- Intake of drugs like non-steroidal anti-inflammatory drugs (NSAIDs) such as ibuprofen, antibiotics, and estrogens.
- Visceral hypersensitivity: This concept states that diseases affecting the gastrointestinal organs 'sensitize' or alter

the responsiveness of the sensory nerves or the processing centres to sensations coming from the organ. According to this theory, a disease such as colitis (inflammation of the colon) can cause permanent changes in the sensitivity of the nerves or processing centres of the colon. As a result of this prior inflammation, normal stimuli are perceived as abnormal (for example, as being painful). Thus, a normal colonic contraction may be painful.

- Small intestinal bacterial overgrowth which can be diagnosed by hydrogen breath testing.
- Diseases like anxiety and depression.

Common symptoms

With indigestion, there are certain symptoms that one must look out for:

- Decreased appetite.
- Pain in the upper abdomen.
- Upper abdominal fullness.
- Feeling of fullness earlier than expected when eating.
- Bloating.
- Belching.
- Nausea (with or without vomiting).
- Heartburn.

Types

There are two kinds of indigestion. The first is Functional dyspepsia/non-ulcer dyspepsia. This is without any evidence of an organic disease that is likely to explain the symptoms. The second kind of indigestion is called Undifferentiated dyspepsia/ non-functional dyspepsia-H.Pylori infection.

WHEN SHOULD ONE SEE A DOCTOR?

One should see a doctor only if consuming meals is becoming increasingly difficult and the symptoms of acidity have been persistent over time.

Prevention

- Indigestion can easily be cured at home if you follow a few easy steps. The best means to prevent indigestion is to consume only those foods that are soft and easy to digest. This will reduce the amount of work that the digestive tract needs to exert. Some people may experience relief from indigestion by eating several small, low-fat meals throughout the day at a slow pace, and by refraining from smoking and abstaining from coffee, carbonated beverages, and alcohol.
- Stopping the use of medications that may irritate the stomach lining—such as aspirin or anti-inflammatory drugs—getting enough rest, and finding ways to decrease emotional and physical stress such as relaxation therapy or yoga are also effective means to keep indigestion at bay.
- Drinking a good quantity of water (an average of 6–8 glasses per day) facilitates healthy digestion.
- Sleep with your head at least 6 inches higher than your chest. You can do this by placing an extra pillow beneath your head. This will keep the digestive juices within the stomach and prevent them from going up the oesophagus.
- Refrain from lying down right after eating.
- Avoid exercising or any strenuous activity after a meal. It is far better to keep an interval of at least an hour between exercise and a meal.

- Reduce alcohol consumption, because alcohol can irritate the lining of the stomach.
- In order to avoid compressing the stomach and restricting its activity, steer clear of tight-fitting garments.
- Cut down on foods with high acid content such as citrus fruits.
- Learn to adapt and to properly cope with stress.

Holistic approach

Digestive symptoms arise as a result of lifestyle, dietary habits, stress, genetic reasons, and some medications. The exact reason has to be assessed before treating the case. For this a holistic evaluation is done. Based on the information, treatments from various disciplines can be suggested. Dietary modifications and yogic postures which aim at strengthening the system help. Internal medications to alter the function and to aid proper digestion are also advised.

Homeopathy

Homeopathic medicines like Nux Vomica, Pulsatilla, Carbo Veg, and China are useful in curing acidity.

Naturopathy

Naturopathic treatments like Vamana Dhouthi, hip baths, and abdominal packs help in curing indigestion.

Ayurveda

Ayurvedic treatments like Choorna Swedam, and internal medications like Hinguvachadi Gulika, Indukantham Kashayam, Jeerakarishtam, and Pippalyasavam are prescribed.

Yoga

Yogasanas like Padahastasana, Vakrasana, Chandra Nadi Prayanama, and relaxation technique also keep the digestive system in order.

Diet

- Maintain regular timings for meals.
- Reduce consumption of fatty and oily food, grilled food, fried food, and junk food.
- Meals should be cut down into small servings so as to make it easier for the stomach to digest.
- The best types of food for bouts of indigestion are fresh fruits and vegetables, especially those that are rich in fibre. Make sure you avoid acidic fruits high in citrus content.
- Try to eat a diet of natural whole foods such as fruits, vegetables, whole grains, meats, nuts, legumes, eggs, and yogurt.
- Avoid carbonated drinks as well as caffeine-rich beverages like coffee.
- Stick with foods that contain liquid and refrain from eating solid foods.

Kitchen cures

- Fasting completely for one day is an efficient method to improve digestion. Taking fruits, fruit juices, and boiled vegetables for one week is a beneficial way of fasting.
- Lemon juice mixed in warm water taken three times a day improves digestion.
- Chewing a small piece of fresh ginger with salt, 5–10 times before meals, stimulates digestion.
- Take equal amounts of ginger powder, black pepper, dried mint leaves, asafoetida (hing), anise seeds, coriander seeds, cumin, fennel, and common salt. Grind together to make a fine powder. Dosage: Take about 1 teaspoon of this powder with water twice a day after meals.
- Drinking buttermilk after a meal improves digestion. Roasted cumin seeds and a little salt in the buttermilk enhances its effectiveness.

- Drinking water gives immediate relief to symptoms like wind, distended stomach, and acidity.
- Eat half a teaspoon of aniseed to improve digestion.
- A teaspoon of ginger juice mixed in a quarter cup of warm water can be taken two or three times a day. A teaspoon of lemon juice and a pinch of salt can also be added to make it more effective.
- Combine a teaspoon of lemon juice, a teaspoon of ginger juice, and two teaspoons of honey. Mix well and consume.
- Add a teaspoon of cumin seeds to warm water and consume the mixture after straining.
- Extract the juice from a teaspoon of coriander leaves, add some salt, and drink twice daily. Coriander juice may also be added to fresh buttermilk to cure indigestion.
- Cinnamon water may also be consumed an hour after meals to ease digestion.
- Herbal teas such as ginger, lavender, raspberry, and chamomile are known to help in easing stomach problems.
- Add mint essence to water and consume every three hours. Mint juice may even be added to honey and lemon juice.
- Make a mixture of 5–6 basil (tulsi) leaves, ¼ teaspoon sea salt, and some black pepper in 3 tablespoons of curd, and then consume it. Repeat this 4 times a day for one week for total reconditioning of the stomach.

DR MATHAI'S TIPS

- To avoid indigestion, it is important to do some light physical activity such as taking a light walk after meals.
- One must also never lie down or sleep immediately after a meal.

- Do at least 30 minutes of brisk walking daily. Also include adequate exercise in the morning to improve the metabolism.
- Do not play active sports immediately after any meal.

Acidity

Gunita Sahni is the Creative Director of a leading television show in Mumbai. In her late 20s, she is up for late hours on shoots, supervizing fellow actors and technicians to make sure everything is perfect. She knows that in today's cut-throat world of television, attaining consistent TRPs for the show is important to keep the producers happy and the money rolling in. But hectic shooting hours made her forget all about sleep or eating. She would get an occasional wink of sleep every now and then between breaks and the pav bhaji from the local street vendor stationed next to their sets has become a staple meal for her over the years.

Last year when she paid me a visit, she was suffering from discomfort and pain in the abdomen. She told me that she had a history of belching, nausea, and complained of a constant bitter taste in her mouth. When the pain was of more severe nature, it would also be accompanied by vomiting and a loss of appetite. Her condition would invariably get worse after eating spicy food, chicken, and meat. Consuming cold milk did ease her pain for a little while, otherwise she would have to take a medicine twice to just get through the day. She was in complete distress.

Whenever there is a history of loss of sleep or alcohol, the chance of acidity increases. After a brief session with Gunita,

I found out that irregular eating timings due to a hectic work schedule and insufficient sleep were the main causes of her problem. I modified her diet and brought subtle changes in her lifestyle so that it suited both her schedule and body. And with a few months of homeopathic medicines and relaxation and breathing exercises, her acidity was taken care of.

Causes

- Malfunctioning of the digestive system.
- Excessive intake of alcohol.
- Acidity also arises either by keeping the stomach empty for a long time or skipping breakfast.
- Eating foods rich in fats like chocolates.
- Pregnancy, ageing, or obesity.
- Eating junk and oily food also leads to burning sensation in stomach and chest area.
- Aspirin and anti-inflammatory drugs.
- Inappropriate food habits.
- Intake of incompatible food.
- Intake of contaminated food.
- Irregular diet.
- Intake of too much sour and spicy food.
- Excessive drinking of tea, coffee, and aerated drinks.
- Smoking.
- Common in patients suffering from liver diseases especially cirrhosis of the liver.
- Helicobacter Pylori infection.
- Eating more food than one's capacity to digest.
- Psychological factors like tension, anxiety, depression, and anger are also considered to trigger the onset of acidity.

Common symptoms

- Burning sensation or pain in the stomach after one to two hours of a meal.

- Constant hunger pangs.
- Constant pain in upper abdomen.
- Belching, nausea, and sometimes vomiting.
- Bitter taste in the mouth.
- Heartburn—characterized by a deeply placed, burning pain in the chest behind the sternum (breast bone).
- It occurs after meals and is precipitated by increase in intra-abdominal pressure like straining or lifting weights.
- Throat dryness in some people.
- Coughing due to acid reflux which causes irritation in throat. In severe cases, this may cause chronic inflammation sensation in throat as well.

Types

In ayurveda, amalpitta or acidity has been described as being of two types. The first is Urdhawaga Amalpitta (with upward pressure, for eg: oesophagitis). The symptoms of Urdhawaga (upward) Amalpitta include vomiting of green, yellow, or slightly red sour fluid which is followed by phlegm; vomiting occurring during digestion of food or due to an empty stomach with occasional bitter or sour taste; belching of similar nature; burning sensation in the throat, chest and upper abdomen; headache; feeling of great heat; loss of appetite; and circular itching studded with numerous small vesicles on the skin.

The second type of acidity in ayurveda is Adhoga Amalpitta (with downward pressure effecting organs like pylorus, duodenum). The symptoms of Adhoga (downward) Amalpitta are thirst, burning sensation, fainting, giddiness, delusion, diarrhoea, occasional oppression in the chest, rashes on the skin, poor digestion, perspiration, and yellowish skin.

Prevention

How many of us have been tempted to go for that offer at a pizza joint where you get two medium pizzas served with unlimited refills of the aerated drinks of your choice? Acidity is a common condition born out of lifestyle stress. A poor diet and lack of sleep makes it much worse. Simple changes in lifestyle can keep the acidity away.

- Skip the aerated drinks as well as the caffeine. Opt for herbal tea instead.
- Have your last meal at least two to three hours before you hit the bed. Keeping long intervals between meals is another cause for acidity. Have small but regular meals. Chew food properly while eating. The saliva generated helps move food through the oesophagus, easing symptoms of heartburn. Also, avoid watching TV or reading books and newpapers while eating food.
- Include vegetables like drumsticks, beans, pumpkin, cabbage, carrots, and spring onions in your diet.
- Prevention mainly consists of avoiding known causative factors like alcohol, spicy foods, drugs like NSAID's, and steroids. Patients with highly nervous and emotional disposition and those involved in high-stress jobs must be given psychological support. Avoiding non-vegetarian foods is also useful in minimizing symptoms of acidity. Moderating lifestyle to include relaxing techniques can go a long way in preventing excess stomach acid and ulcers.
- Try to identify foods that contribute to excess stomach acid as it may vary from person to person. Foods that are spicy, salty, and acidic should generally be avoided.
- Smoking and alcohol consumption should be stopped to keep stomach acid levels in the stomach and oesophagus in harmony.
- Eat regular meals and follow a healthy diet.
- Take extra care when lifting weights, as this puts the abdominal area under added strain and may result in digestion problems.

Holistic approach

The approach is to correct the digestive system, to regulate acid secretion, to strengthen the gastric mucosa, and to make dietary changes to prevent ulcer formation.

Homeopathy

Homeopathic medicines like Nux Vomica, Pusatilla, Carbo Veg, and China are good for acidity.

Naturopathy

Naturopathic treatments like abdominal packs or local mud applications to abdomen and kidney packs help in acidity.

Ayurveda

Ayurvedic medicines help in treatment of acidity and making the person's constitution stronger.

Treatments like Snehapanam, Virechanam, Vasti and medications like Sankha Bhasma, Amrutharishtam, Indukantham Kashayam, and Madiphala Rasayanam help.

Yoga

Stretching exercises including yogasanas. Yogasanas like Padahastasana, Vakrasana, and Chandra Nadi Pranayama help in combating and reducing acidity.

Diet

- Eat fruits like apples, watermelons, and bananas. Avoid fried food, pickles, and hot and spicy food. Take your meals on time. Drink plenty of water. Don't skip your meals. Include lots of vegetables in your diet. Eat light meals that make it easy for the digestive system to quickly digest the food you eat.
- Habits: Smoking and alcohol consumption must be stopped.
- Exercise: Daily brisk walks for half an hour in the mornings.

Kitchen cures

- ❖ Drinking buttermilk helps control acidity. You can add ginger to the buttermilk.
- ❖ Eat curd rice at least once a day.
- ❖ Drink one glass of ragi porridge in the morning. This helps in reducing acidity.
- ❖ Drinking half a glass of cold milk has a cooling effect on the stomach.
- ❖ Mint (pudina) juice is also a good medicine for acidity.
- ❖ Tender coconut water had on an empty stomach gives a cooling effect and relieves acidity.
- ❖ Drinking ash gourd juice on an empty stomach gives relief from hyper acidity and cures ulcers.
- ❖ Bananas makes a good coating on the mucosal linings of the stomach and relieve acidity.
- ❖ Indian gooseberry is a good remedy for acidity.
- ❖ Eating basil leaves or cucumber in the morning helps to get rid of acidity.
- ❖ Concentrated lemon juice helps to overcome acidity. Lemon contains potassium which reduces acid and helps in easy digestion.
- ❖ Cumin seeds, coriander, sugar candy powdered in equal quantities and taken 2 spoonfuls twice a day also helps to cure acidity.
- ❖ Half a spoon of black pepper (kali mirch) powder taken with rock salt twice a day helps to get relief from acidity as well.

DR MATHAI'S TIPS

- ❖ Bananas have defensive action against acidity and heartburn.

- Stay away from fried foods, pickles, hot spicy foods, vinegar, and chocolate.
- Drink lots of water, at least 8 glasses each day.
- Drink a glass of cold milk for quick relief of heartburn and acidity.
- Boiled ash gourd with jaggery relieves bloating and burning sensation in stomach associated with acidity and gastritis.
- Add one tablespoon of triphala powder to one glass of water, boil, and reduce to half a glass and filter. This hot water decoction, along with one tablespoon of honey or ghee, relieves gastritis.
- Drink water soaked with coriander seeds or jeera seeds—it's an effective remedy for acidity.

ULCERS

Shweta, a mid-30s housewife residing in Dwarka, New Delhi, loves eating spicy food. Her kitchen larders are always stocked with a large supply of spicy potato chips and namkeens. Cooking food without the generous pinch of red mirch is a complete no-no for her and her husband's repeated complaints of the food being too spicy falls on deaf ears. Shweta chooses to remain oblivious to the side effects of eating too much spicy food than give up on them. Then one day, she was shocked to see blood in her morning stool. This proved to be the turning point for Shweta. She decided to take stock of the situation and came to me for treatment.

Shweta was a worried woman when she visited me. Spotting blood in her stool had shaken her out of her state of complacency and she was ready to do anything to get her body back on track. She complained of severe stomach pain, bloating, coating of the tongue, reflux, and irritation of the throat. Prescription of a few homeopathic medicines and counselling has substantially reduced the ulcers.

Causes

- The direct cause of peptic ulcers is the destruction of the gastric or intestinal mucosal lining by hydrochloric acid, an acid normally present in the digestive juices of the stomach.
- Infection with the bacterium Helicobactor Pylori is thought to play an important role in causing both gastric and duodenal ulcers. Helicobacter Pylori may be transmitted from person to person through contaminated food and water.
- Injury of the gastric mucosa and weakening of the mucous defenses are also responsible for gastric ulcers. Excess secretion of hydrochloric acid, genetic predisposition, and psychological stress are important contributing factors in the formation and worsening of duodenal ulcers.
- Chronic use of anti-inflammatory medications, such as aspirin.
- Smoking.
- Excessive alcohol consumption.
- Improper diet, irregular, or skipped meals.
- Stress does not cause an ulcer, but may be a contributing factor.
- Chronic disorders such as liver disease, emphysema, and rheumatoid arthritis may increase vulnerability to ulcers.

Common symptoms

The major symptom of an ulcer is burning or gnawing feeling in the stomach area that lasts between 30 minutes to 3 hours. This pain is often interpreted as hunger. The pain usually occurs in the upper abdomen. In some individuals the pain occurs immediately after eating and in others the pain may not occur until hours after eating. Sometimes frequent pain can awaken the person at night. Pain can be relieved by drinking milk, eating, resting, or taking antacids. Other symptoms include:

- Loss of appetite.
- Weight loss.
- Persons with duodenal ulcers may experience weight gain because the person eats more to ease discomfort.
- Recurrent vomiting, blood in the stool, and anaemia are other symptoms.

Types

Ulcers can be of five different kinds. The first is Gastric Ulcer which occurs in the stomach. Then is Duodenal Ulcer which is present in the duodenum. The third kind of ulcer is Oesophageal Ulcer which occurs in the lower end of oesophagus. Oesophageal ulcers are often associated with a bad case of acid reflux, or GERD. Bleeding Ulcer is one which causes internal bleeding as a result of having been left untreated. And last is Refractory Ulcer which heals after at least 3 months of treatment.

Prevention

- Eat food at proper time and do not skip meals.
- Avoid spicy and sour food.
- Avoid smoking and alcohol.
- Do not have tea and coffee on an empty stomach.
- Manage stress effectively.

For a person suffering from ulcers, the most important thing to keep in mind is that he/she should neither indulge in food nor avoid food. There should always be a healthy balance in food intake. A lot of times, people are in a hurry to eat, so they don't chew their food well before intake. Another very important thing is that one should know how to manage stress when such situations arise. Make sure to include more raw food like fresh fruits and green leafy vegetables in your diet. Restrict the intake of caffeine, citrus products, and sodas and avoid smoking and alcohol.

Holistic approach

The approach is to correct the digestive system, to regulate acid secretion, to strengthen the gastric mucosa, and to make dietary changes to cure ulcers and to prevent it in future.

Homeopathy

Homeopathic medicines like Nux Vomica, Argentum Nitricum, Anacardium, Kali Bichromicum, Phosphorus, and Graphites are some of the constitutional medicines for ulcers in the digestive track.

Naturopathy

Naturopathic relaxation techniques, hip baths, and abdominal packs help in treating ulcers. Deep breathing exercises help in relieving stress. Above all, the patient must try to rid himself of worries and stay cheerful. He should also cultivate regularity in his habits of work, exercise, or rest. Drink at least 6–8 glasses of fresh water in a day. Tea made out of fenugreek seeds is very effective in treating ulcers.

Ayurveda

According to ayurveda, ulcers are often linked to an imbalance in Pitta. Treatment includes dietary and lifestyle changes.

It is considered to be the effect of deranged Pitta. So, all the treatments and medications aim at balancing it. Treatments like Vasti, and Virechana are helpful along with Abhyanga and Sirodhara.

Internal medications like Kashayams, medicated ghee, and tablets are also prescribed.

Yoga
Yogasanas like Chandra Nadi Pranayama and Brahmari Pranayama help.

Kitchen cures
- Ash gourd juice to be taken first thing in the morning.
- Soak bael leaves in warm water for 20 minutes and drink on empty stomach, or eat fully ripened bale fruit in the morning.
- Banana neutralizes the acidic nature of the stomach and reduces ulcers.
- Cabbage is regarded as another useful home remedy for ulcer. Boil cabbage in water till the water reduces to half the quantity and take twice a day.

Constipation

Constipation is something that has affected almost everyone of us at one time or another. Take the case of Rachita Sodhi, a Delhi-based fashion designer whose prêt designer boutique in Hauz Khas village caters to the city's elite. Recently separated from her husband, she lives alone with her 2-year-old daughter. With the Delhi glitterati lining up for her outfits, she is as busy as one could be. But only Rachita knows what it takes to run the boutique all day long, especially during the festive season when the demand for her designer clothes shoots up. Reprimanding tailors at the workshop is part and parcel of her routine. But there is another Rachita to her besides the strong-minded business lady—the one crying from constipation in the bathroom every second day.

On meeting me, Rachita said that she had been suffering from constipation since childhood. She complained of having very hard stools, saying how passing them is very painful for her, sometimes even leading to bleeding from her anus. Looking at her eating patterns, I saw that constipation arose at around the time she would consume more meat and carbohydrates, and also after her periods. Additionally to her constipation, her hands would always tremble. She was short tempered and her BP used to shoot up very often. Adding to her woes, she was also overweight. Having been divorced recently, she had a lot of fear and anxiety, leading to a lack of sleep. She was put on homeopathic and ayurvedic medicines and was given counselling sessions to help her deal with the separation better. Her condition gradually improved and she still continues her treatment under my care.

Constipation is defined as having a bowel movement fewer than three times per week. But even people who have bowel movements daily and fail to get one also claim to be constipated. With constipation, stools are usually hard, dry, small in size, and difficult to eliminate. Some people who are constipated find it painful to have a bowel movement and often experience straining, bloating, and the sensation of a full bowel.

Many people think they are constipated when, in fact, their bowel movements are regular. A medical history and physical exam may be the only diagnostic tests needed before the doctor suggests treatment.

Constipation is a symptom, not a disease. Almost everyone experiences constipation at some point in their life, and a poor diet typically is the cause. Most of the times, constipation is temporary and not serious. Understanding its causes, prevention, and treatment will help most people find relief.

Causes

To understand constipation, it helps to know how the colon, or the large intestine, works. As food moves through the colon, the colon absorbs water from the food while it forms waste products, or stool. Muscle contractions in the colon then push the stool toward the rectum. By the time stool reaches the rectum it is solid, because most of the water has been absorbed.

Constipation occurs when the colon absorbs too much water or if the colon's muscle contractions are slow or sluggish, causing the stool to move through the colon too slowly. As a result, stools can become hard and dry. Common causes of constipation are

- ❖ Not enough fibre in the diet.
- ❖ Not enough liquids.
- ❖ Lack of physical activity.
- ❖ Medications.

The most common causes of constipation are poor diet and lack of exercise. Other causes of constipation include medications, irritable bowel syndrome, abuse of laxatives, and specific diseases.

Some medications can cause constipation, including,

- ❖ Pain medications (especially narcotics).
- ❖ Antacids that contain aluminum and calcium.
- ❖ Blood pressure medications (calcium channel blockers).
- ❖ Antiparkinson drugs.
- ❖ Antispasmodics.
- ❖ Antidepressants.
- ❖ Iron supplements.
- ❖ Diuretics.
- ❖ Anticonvulsants.

Intestinal obstructions, scar tissue—also called adhesions—diverticulosis, tumours, colorectal stricture, Hirschsprung disease, or cancer can compress, squeeze, or narrow the intestine and rectum and also cause constipation.

Consequences

Sometimes constipation can lead to complications. These complications include haemorrhoids, caused by straining to have a bowel movement, or anal fissures—tears in the skin around the anus—caused when hard stool stretches the sphincter muscle. As a result, rectal bleeding may occur, appearing as bright red streaks on the surface of the stool.

At times straining causes a small amount of intestinal lining to push out from the anal opening. This condition, known as rectal prolapse, may lead to secretion of mucus from the anus. Usually eliminating the cause of the prolapse, such as straining or coughing, is the only treatment necessary.

Constipation may also cause hard stool to pack the intestine and rectum so tightly that the normal pushing action of the colon is not enough to expel the stool. This condition, called faecal impaction, occurs most often in children and older adults.

Lifestyle causes

- Lack of fibre/liquids in the diet: Fibre, both soluble and insoluble, is a part of fruits, vegetables, and grains that the body cannot digest. Soluble fibre dissolves easily in water and takes on a soft, gel-like texture in the intestines. Insoluble fibre passes through the intestines almost unchanged. The bulk and soft texture of fibre helps prevent hard, dry stool that is difficult to pass. Liquids add fluid to the colon and bulk to stools, making bowel movements softer and easier to pass. People who have problems with constipation should try to drink liquids every day. However, liquids that contain caffeine, such as coffee and cola drinks, will worsen one's symptoms by causing dehydration. Alcohol is another beverage that causes dehydration.

- Lack of physical activity: Lack of physical activity is thought to be one of the reasons why constipation is common in older people.
- Changes in life or routine.
- Pregnancy.
- Travelling.
- Ageing may also affect bowel regularity, because a slower metabolism results in less intestinal activity and muscle tone.
- Abuse of laxatives: Although people may feel relief when they use laxatives, typically they must increase the dose over time because the body grows reliant on laxatives in order to have a bowel movement. As a result, laxatives may become habit-forming.
- People who ignore the urge to have a bowel movement may eventually stop feeling the need to have one, which can lead to constipation. Children may postpone having a bowel movement because of stressful toilet training or because they do not want to interrupt their play. Adults ignore the urge because of emotional stress or because they are busy.
- Specific diseases: Diseases that cause constipation include neurological disorders, metabolic and endocrine disorders, and systemic conditions that affect organ systems.
- Neurological disorders like multiple sclerosis, Parkinson's disease, chronic idiopathic intestinal pseudo-obstruction, stroke, and spinal cord injuries.
- Metabolic and endocrine conditions like diabetes, uremia, hypercalcaemia, poor glycemic control, and hypothyroidism.
- Systemic disorders like amyloidosis, lupus, and scleroderma.
- Problems with the colon and rectum: Intestinal obstruction, diverticulosis, tumours, colorectal stricture, Hirschsprung disease, or cancer of colon can compress, squeeze, or narrow the intestine and rectum and cause constipation.

Common symptoms

- Adults with constipation may feel bloating, headache, hard stools, difficulty in passing stools, and sometimes bleeding while passing stools.
- Children with constipation may strain, cry, draw legs towards abdomen, or arch the back while having a bowel movement.

Types

The two types of constipation are Idiopathic Constipation and Functional Constipation. Irritable bowel syndrome (IBS) with predominant symptoms of constipation is categorized separately. Idiopathic Constipation is of unknown origin. Functional Constipation means that the bowel is healthy but not working properly. Functional constipation is often the result of poor dietary habits and lifestyle. It occurs in both children and adults and is most common in women.

When should you see a doctor?

You need to see a doctor if your home remedies fail or you have the following complaints.

- **Abdominal constipation symptoms:** If you have constipation symptoms such as cramps or abdominal pains, then it is possible that you have a blockage or faecal impaction. The impaction generally forms at the bottom of your intestines and rectum. The longer the faecal impaction remains, the more severe and intense the constipation symptoms will become. Toxins and bacteria will begin to flood back into the body and cause serious infections.
- **Bloody constipation symptoms:** Constipation symptoms involving blood in the stool may also be caused by rectal bleeding. Rectal bleeding can be caused by fissures which are the result of dry, hard stool tearing the anal tissue

during a bowel movement. Blood in the stool is one of those constipation symptoms that really require a physician's attention because it may be the result of polyps or colon cancer.

Prevention

Although treatment depends on the cause, severity, and duration of the constipation, in most cases dietary and lifestyle changes will help relieve symptoms and help prevent them from recurring.

- Diet: A diet with enough fibre helps the body form soft, bulky stool. High-fibre foods include beans, whole grains and bran cereals, fresh fruits, and vegetables such as asparagus, brussels sprouts, cabbage, and carrots. For people prone to constipation, limiting foods that have little or no fibre, such as ice cream, cheese, meat, and processed foods is also important.
- Supplementation: Supplementation with magnesium and large doses of Vitamin-C have a mild laxative effect on the body.
- Water: Drink plenty of water, especially if you are taking supplemental fibre.
- Lifestyle changes: Other changes that may help treat and prevent constipation include drinking other liquids such as fruit and vegetable juices and clear soups, engaging in daily exercise, and reserving enough time to have a bowel movement. In addition, the urge to have a bowel movement should not be ignored.
- Exercise daily.
- Reduce stress level: This help the body to relax. This can help relax the colon.

Holistic approach

Holistic approach mainly includes diet regulation by adopting a fibre-rich food diet and proper lifestyle. Naturopathic therapies like Enema, hip baths, colonic irrigation, local abdominal massages, GH packs, kidney packs, and mud application also help in curing constipation. Yogic techniques like Shanka Prakshalana, abdominal asanas, mudras and bandhas along with internal ayurvedic medication also go a long way.

Homoeopathy

Homeopathic philosophy lays great stress on leading an active and healthy lifestyle while treating such diseases. The prescription depends upon symptoms or the causative factors of the constipation. Medicines like Nux Vomica, Bryonia, Alumina, Magnesium Muriaticum are some of the remedies that are useful in treating constipation.

Nux Vomica is a good remedy for constipation with an unsatisfactory feeling. Bryonia is for constipation with hard stools which are very dry and difficult to pass. Calcarea Carb and Silicea are other remedies for obstinate constipation. These are to be taken in consultation with a homeopathic doctor.

Naturopathy

Treatments like hip baths and abdomen compress help relieve constipation. Simply drinking lots of water also helps relieve constipation. Naturopathy believes in making dietary changes and in regulation of bowels through exercises—mainly yoga.

1. Enema: plain water enema is the quickest remedy for constipation. Usually used as quick relief for obstinate constipation.
2. Colonic irrigation.
3. Neutral hip bath: It comprises of the person sitting in a tub of water at room temperature, immersing the parts between the ribs and thighs into water.

4. Abdominal packs and compresses either with mud or cold water applied on the abdomen.

Ayurveda

According to ayurveda, constipation is mostly caused due to aggravation of Vata (air), though high Pitta and Kapha doshas can also contribute in some of the cases. Specialized ayurvedic medications can be taken under prescription of an ayurvedic physician. Vata pacifying treatments and treatments to improve oleation like Abhyanga, Vasti, herbal hip baths, and internal medications to improve digestion and excretion like Triphala, Kalyanagulam, Manibhadragulam, Hingutriguna Tailam, Gandharvahasta Tailam, Gandharvahastadi Kashayam, Chiruvilwadi Kashayam are all used.

Diet containing fibre, oily foods, and easily digestible foods is recommended.

Yoga

Asanas that are beneficial to cure constipation areVajrasana, Vakrasana, Ushtrasana, Pawanmuktasana, Baddha Konasana and Makarabhyasa.

Diet

The diet should include whole grains, flour with bran, high-fibre vegetables like gourds and leafy vegetables, fruits especially bulk forming fruits like papaya, melons, and dry fruits like dates, figs, prunes, and black raisins.

Kitchen cures

- Guava and its seeds provide necessary fibre to diet and thus help to relieve constipation.
- Add fruits such as pears, grapes, orange juice, and papaya to the diet to overcome constipation.
- Add a little sugar or honey to a glass of milk and drink it twice a day.

- Another home remedy to regulate bowel movement is to eat raisins on a regular basis. Soak 6–8 raisins in hot water. Crush them when they become cool and then consume.
- Ginger tea is an effective home remedy for constipation. It facilitates bowel movement.
- If badly needed, natural laxatives like husks of Isabgol can be taken.
- Include spinach in your diet.

Anorexia

I once had a patient named Tanya who had come complaining of sagging breasts. Ever since childhood, Tanya had been conscious of how she looked and could not tolerate putting on even a single extra kilo on her body. She would be under constant peer pressure of losing weight and staying thin. She got married when she was merely 20. Blessed with a baby girl soon after the marriage, she worked hard to get her pre-pregnancy shape back after delivery. A new mother needs to rest for a few months after delivery, but Tanya ignored all that in her pursuit to reach the desired weight. This ultimately wreaked havoc on her body. She had put on weight after delivery and had again lost weight by severe exercise and changes in her diet. She also suffered from flatulence and headaches. A few homeopathic medicines, counselling, chest exercises, and yoga were helpful in treating her condition.

As anorexia is more of a psychological and behavioural disorder, I advise psychological counselling for achievement of complete cure. The mental aspect of anorexia is a hindrance in the path of treatment. Friends and family must provide emotional support to such patients.

Causes

Anorexia can arise due to a mix of social, emotional, and biological factors.

- Psychological: People with anorexia are often overachievers and perfectionists. They focus on pleasing others and feeling helpless and unhappy inside. Low self-confidence with perfectionism is a combination that can push someone to anorexia.
- Social: Societal and family pressure to be thin can also contribute to anorexia.
- Biological: It is found that anorexia sometimes runs in families.

Common symptoms

- Marked weight loss.
- Fear of getting fat even when underweight.
- Denial of hunger with obsession of counting calories.
- Excessive exercise.
- Frequent weighing.
- Constipation.
- Dry sallow skin.
- Loss of stamina.
- Thinning of hair due to lack of proper nutrition.
- Fainting spells.

When should you see a doctor?

Consult a doctor when you or someone in the family are having the following symptoms:

- Rapid weight loss.
- Eating very little and being overtly concerned about weight and appearance.
- See yourself as fat and feel that you must diet, even when other people say you look too thin.

- Not having regular periods.
- Feel the need to exercise a lot, and do not give yourself healing or rest time when you are injured or exhausted.

Prevention

- Children need to be fed with positive body images, especially girls.
- Watch teens carefully. Encourage them to be more active.
- Provide a non-judgmental ear to the child when it comes to discussing fears or anxieties.
- Do not make fun of anybody's body image.

Holistic approach

Holistic treatment programmes aim to heal the body, mind, and spirit. Healthy lifestyles, eating plans, and sporting activities promote wellness and recovery from eating disorders.

Homeopathy

Homeopathic medicines including Lycopodium, Natrum Muriaticum, Nux Vomica, and Arsenicum Album are some of the constitutional medicines which help in treating anorexia.

Naturopathy

Naturopathic treatments like spinal baths, head and neck acupressure, reflexology, and eye packs help in treating anorexia.

Ayurveda

The ayurvedic treatment of anorexia is aimed at achieving weight gain and correcting the distorted thinking and self-image of persons affected with this disorder. It is also important to prevent complications resulting from this condition, which can prove to be serious or life-threatening. Ayurvedic medicines improve appetite and help in digestion of food.

Healing activities such as yoga and meditation help patients to focus and remain calm in their battle against this destructive illnesses.

Yoga

Yogasanas include basic stretching exercises, Brahmari Pranayama, and meditation techniques.

Kitchen cures

- Take two or three cloves and boil them with a cup of water. Add juice of half lime and divide the preparation in two halves and drink it twice a day.
- Every day during breakfast have two or three oranges or one glass of orange juice to sharpen the appetite.
- Apples are a useful remedy for anorexia. Eat 2 fresh apples every day. There are enzymes in the stomach for digestion of food. Active ingredients of the apples will stimulate the flow of enzymes for improved digestion.
- Mix ginger with lime juice and add rock salt to taste. Keep this preparation in sunlight for 3 days. Taking one teaspoon after every meal will enhance the capacity of the digestive system.

DR MATHAI'S TIPS

- Prevention is very important in anorexia. Avoid intake of oily or spicy food.
- Develop the habit of mild exercising. Exercise will improve the digestion and it will also help digestive system to grasp every bit of vitamins and minerals available in the food.

- Restore normal body health with a combination of various vegetables and fresh fruits. Once the body retains its normal health, recovery will be much faster.

BULEMIA

Ashna Tewari is on her way to enrol her name in a beauty pageant. All of 16, she hopes her age won't be a deterrent to her participation. Making her way to the pageant head office in a taxi, she applies another quote of the red lipstick purchased on the sly. Her little black dress paired with fishnet stockings are enough to make the guard mistake her for an adult and usher her in. Unable to produce a proof of age, Ashna is ultimately shown the door by the judges.

In a country where young girls are fed on pictures of size-zero heroines, bulimia is an all too common problem. These girls, mostly teenagers, are so obsessed with body image and weight that they don't realize it may have an adverse effect on their social, emotional, and physical well-being.

I get patients like Ashna all the time in my clinic. One particular lady came to me with indigestion, stomach pain, and digestive issues. She kept on complaining about how ugly she was and hated the way she looked even though no one could see anything wrong in her physical appearance. On further examination, it was found that her throat was congested, almost as if it had been scratched. She finally admitted to having bulimia. The approach, constitutional homeopathic medicines, and counselling helped restore her life back to normal over a period of time.

Causes

- Bulimia occurs when a person is unhappy with the way they look, and develops over time. It can occur together with other psychiatric disorders such as depression, obsessive-compulsive disorder, substance dependence, or self-injurious behaviour, post-traumatic stress disorder and some personality disorders.
- There may be some genetic factor to developing bulimia, which is triggered by stressful or traumatic life experiences. For example, some people with bulimia have had a childhood where there were frequent family problems with arguments and criticism at home. Some people with bulimia have been abused as a child.
- A chemical called serotonin which is in parts of the brain is thought to have something to do with bulimia. In some way one or more of the above factors, or even other unknown factors, may lead to a low level of serotonin.

Common symptoms

- Eating uncontrollably.
- Strict dieting.
- Fasting.
- Vigorous exercise.
- Vomiting or abusing laxatives or diuretics in an attempt to lose weight.
- Preoccupation with body weight.
- Depression or mood swings.
- Feeling out of control.
- Swollen glands in neck and face.
- Weakness and exhaustion.

Types

There are two types of bulimia. The first is the purging type in which the person regularly engages in self-induced vomiting or the misuse of laxatives, diuretics, or enemas. The second kind is the non-purging type in which the individual uses fasting or excessive exercise to control weight, but does not regularly purge.

When should you see a doctor?

A doctor needs to be consulted if the child develops signs like lack of control overeating, secrecy in eating, eating unusually large amount of food, alternating between fasting and overeating, and is obsessed with how they look.

Prevention

Early treatment is the best way to prevent progression of the disease. Adults in the family need to help the teens and children to develop healthy view about them and to have a positive attitude.

Holistic approach

Bulimia needs a holistic approach in treatment. Counselling, family counselling, cognitive behaviour therapy to change food, eating, and exercise behaviours, and nutritional planning are necessary and give a holistic approach to treating the entire person. These are very useful for supporting both physical and mental healing.

Homeopathy

Homeopathic medicines like Passiflora Incarnata soothes the mind and calms the nerves. Hypericum Perforatum or St John's Wort has been very successful in treating depression accompanied by an eating disorder. Some other medicines are Argentum Nitricum, Ignatia, Natrum Mur, Pulsatilla, and Staphysagria.

Naturopathy
Naturopathic treatments like Auriculotherapy, abdomen packs, hip baths, and diet counselling help to overcome bulimia.

Ayurveda
Ayurvedic treatments like Sirodhara, Thalam, Abhyangam, Nasyam help in bulimia.

Meditation helps in suspending thought and directing attention in a calm and focused manner.

Yoga
Suryanamaskar and other yogaasanas like Ardha Chakrasana, Ustrasana, Padahastasana Vakrasana, and Bhujangasana help develop slim long muscles, which in turn improve the definition of the body and can help somebody who suffers from bulimia to feel better about the way they look.

Diet
- Diet counselling: Dietary multivitamin supplements, Vitamin B complex with C are needed.
- Bulimic patients may have a zinc deficiency, and zinc is an important mineral needed by the body for normal hormonal activity and enzymatic function.
- Foods rich in zinc are celery, asparagus, borage, figs, potatoes, and eggplants.

Kitchen cures
- Have meals together as a family.
- A great home remedy for bulimia is to eat oranges for easy digestion. People who are suffering from bulimia tend to feel bloated and very heavy after they eat. This is what leads to purging and further sickness. Oranges tend to help move the food through the digestive tract much faster. Try mixing oranges into meals, salad, or desserts.

- Drinking plenty of water can really helps to ease digestion.

DR MATHAI'S TIPS

- Stick to the treatment plan. Don't skip therapy sessions and try not to stray from meal plans even if they make you uncomfortable.
- Get the right nutrition. Talk to the doctor about appropriate vitamin and mineral supplements.
- Learn about bulimia. Education about the condition can empower the person and motivate them to overcome it.
- Don't isolate yourself from caring family members and friends who want to see you get healthy.
- Be kind to yourself. Resist urges to weigh or check in the mirror frequently.

OBESITY

Obesity is a medical condition in which excess body fat accumulates to the extent that it may have an adverse effect on health, leading to reduced life expectancy and/or increased health problems· People are considered obese when their body mass index (BMI), a measure obtained by dividing one's weight in kilograms by the square of one's height in metres, exceeds 30 kg/m^{2}· Obesity increases the likelihood of various diseases, particularly heart disease, type 2 diabetes, obstructive sleep apnea, certain types of cancer, and osteoarthritis.

One of the most painful aspects of obesity may be the emotional suffering it causes. In addition, many people wrongly stereotype obese people as gluttonous, lazy, or both. However, more and more evidence contradicts this assumption. Obese people often face prejudice or discrimination at work, at school, while looking for a job, and in social situations. Feelings of rejection, shame, or depression are common.

Take Arnab Dasgupta's case, for example. A 31-year-old writer from Kolkata, Arnab had always had a weight problem. No matter how carefully he ate or how much exercise he did, he could never beat his weight problem. So much so that after a while he just gave up on the exercising and any other efforts he was putting in. Being overweight is a part of his daily life for him, and includes trouble finding the right kind of clothes, being mocked by people on the streets, having no control over his eating and recently, having trouble getting his book published because the publishers said that he wouldn't look good on the cover. He had recently also discovered that he had high blood pressure and was at risk for diabetes.

When Arnab came to me, apart from having health issues, he was also quite depressed. His constant battle with weight had pulled him down and he was unable to bring himself back up. I spent a lot of time talking to him, understanding his entire life history, his work schedules and lifestyle, and that is a key aspect of treating his obesity.

Obesity is an excess proportion of total body fat. A person is considered obese when his or her weight is 20 percent or more above normal weight. The most common measure of obesity is the body mass index or BMI. A person is considered overweight if the BMI is between 25 and 29.9; a person is considered obese if the BMI is over 30.

Causes

Obesity occurs when a person consumes more calories than he or she burns. For many people this boils down to eating too much and exercising too little. But there are other factors that also play a role in obesity. These may include:

- Age: As you get older, your body's ability to metabolize food slows down and you do not require as many calories to maintain your weight. This is why people often note that while they eat the same quantity and do the same activities as they did when they were 20-years-old, they start gaining weight at age 40.
- Gender: Women tend to be more overweight than men. Men have a higher resting metabolic rate (meaning they burn more energy at rest) than women, so men require more calories to maintain their body weight. Additionally, when women become postmenopausal, their metabolic rate decreases. That is partly why many women gain weight after menopause.
- Genetics: Obesity (and thinness) tends to run in families.
- Environmental factors: Although genes are an important factor in many cases of obesity, a person's environment also plays a significant role. Environmental factors include lifestyle behaviours such as what a person eats and how active he or she is.
- Physical activity: Active individuals require more calories than less active ones to maintain their weight. Additionally, physical activity tends to decrease appetite in obese individuals while increasing the body's ability to preferentially metabolize fat as an energy source.
- Psychological factors: Psychological factors also influence eating habits and obesity. Many people eat in response to negative emotions such as boredom, sadness, or anger. People who have difficulty with weight management may be facing more emotional and psychological issues; about 30 percent of people who seek treatment for serious weight problems have difficulties with binge eating. During a

binge-eating episode, people eat large amounts of food while feeling they can't control how much they are eating.

- Illness: Although not as common as many believe, there are some illnesses that can cause obesity. These include hormone problems such as hypothyroidism (poorly acting thyroid slows metabolism), depression, and some rare diseases of the brain that can lead to overeating.
- Medication: Certain drugs, such as steroids and some antidepressants, may cause excessive weight gain.
- Sedentary lifestyle: Sedentary people burn fewer calories than people who are active.
- Excessive food intake: Overeating leads to weight gain, especially if the diet is high in fat.
- Endocrine disorders, diseases such as hypothyroidism, insulin resistance, polycystic ovarian syndrome, and Cushing's syndrome are also contributors to obesity.
- Medications associated with weight gain include certain antidepressants, anticonvulsants, diabetic medications.
- Certain hormones such as oral contraceptives and most corticosteroids such as prednisone. Weight gain may also be seen with some high blood pressure medications and antihistamines.
- Management is one of the most important key factors in dealing with obesity in long-term. The primary goal of management of obesity should be improvement of obesity related conditions and reduce the risk of developing future diseases. It involves balance of three essential elements of lifestyle: dietary habits, physical activity, and behaviour modification.

When should you see a doctor?

You should call your doctor if you are having emotional or psychological issues related to your obesity or need help losing weight. If your BMI is 30 or greater, you're considered obese. You should talk to your doctor about losing weight since you are at high risk of having health problems.

Complications from obesity

If you're obese, you're more likely to develop a number of potentially serious health problems, including:

- ❖ High cholesterol and triglycerides.
- ❖ Type-2 diabetes.
- ❖ High blood pressure.
- ❖ Metabolic syndrome—a combination of high blood sugar, high blood pressure, high triglycerides, and high cholesterol.
- ❖ Heart disease.
- ❖ Stroke.
- ❖ Cancer, including cancer of the uterus, cervix, ovaries, breast, colon, rectum, and prostate.
- ❖ Sleep apnea, a potentially serious sleep disorder in which breathing repeatedly stops and starts.
- ❖ Depression.
- ❖ Gallbladder disease.
- ❖ Gynaecological problems, such as infertility and irregular periods.
- ❖ Erectile dysfunction and sexual health issues due to deposits of fat blocking or narrowing the arteries to the genitals.
- ❖ Non-alcoholic fatty liver disease, a condition in which fat builds up in the liver and can cause inflammation or scarring.
- ❖ Osteoarthritis.
- ❖ Skin problems, such as poor wound healing.

Quality of life

When you're obese, your overall quality of life may be lower, too. You may not be able to do things you'd normally enjoy as easily as you'd like. You may have trouble participating in family activities. You may avoid public places. You may even encounter discrimination.

Other weight-related issues that may affect your quality of life include:

- Depression
- Disability
- Physical discomfort
- Sexual problems
- Shame
- Social isolation

Prevention

Obesity, as well as other related diseases, are largely preventable. Supportive environments and communities are fundamental in shaping people's choices, making the healthier choice of foods and regular physical activity the easiest choice, and therefore preventing obesity. At the individual level, people can:

- Limit energy intake from total fats.
- Increase consumption of fruit and vegetables, as well as legumes, whole grains, and nuts.
- Limit the intake of sugars.
- Engage in regular physical activity.
- Achieve energy balance and a healthy weight.
- Ensure the availability of healthy food choices and support regular physical activity practice in the workplace.

Holistic approach

Because of the complex nature of obesity, a holistic approach is often identified as the best practice to manage obesity. The imbalances in the patient's overall constitution are at the root of disease and dysfunction, including obesity. Therefore, treatment focused on the person's overall well-being would ultimately address obesity. Holistic treatments for obesity include lifestyle management, dynamic yoga and exercise.

Changes in diet, de-stress and detox programmes (Panchakarma and naturopathic therapies), and medicines (homeopathic/ayurvedic) acupuncture aim to remove the root cause for obesity by improving the metabolism, regulating the digestion, absorption and elimination processes, and reducing the stress levels.

Going on a well-organized yoga program with a detox diet of mainly liquids, fruits, and vegetables improves metabolism and helps in weight loss.

Diet would be advised as per individual needs, after assessing the body, and this helps in maintaining and keeping up with the weight loss.

Homeopathy

Homeopathy not only helps you in losing weight but it improves your metabolism, digestive system, and elementary system. But the medicines need to be individually prescribed, based on your own unique pattern of symptoms. There are many reasons for weight issues like hypothyroidism, genetic factors, and hormonal imbalances. The underlying cause of the weight is analyzed by complete homeopathic evaluation and medicines are given accordingly.

Naturopathy

Naturopathy considers obesity to be less about diet and more about correcting underlying imbalances through lifestyle changes that requires a plan of care that supports long-term sustainable health optimization. Teaching patients how to eat, exercise, and relax/nurture themselves physically and emotionally is crucial to treatment. Treatments such as deep tissue massages, underwater massages, jet baths, steam baths, Turkish baths, plantain leaf baths, and full mud baths help reduce weight.

Ayurvedic and homeopathic internal medications are targeted at the cause for the condition and are adviced likewise.

Dietary changes help a lot along with regular strict exercise pattern. Carbohydrates and fats should be reduced and one should include vegetables, proteins, fish, and chicken without skin.

Ayurveda

Diet, exercise, internal medications, and external treatments should be administered judiciously to manage obesity.

Treatments like Choorna Swedam and Udvarthanam reduce Kapha and mobilize fat. Teekshna Vasti is important. Medicines like Varnadi Kashayam, Guggulutiktha Kashayam, Yavaloha Choornam, Kokum extract, Vidangam, Devadaru, and Yavam are all helpful medicines. Sleep during the day should be strictly avoided. Other ayurvedic treatments like Patrapotala Swedam, and Dhanyamlaswedam help lose weight and tone the muscles.

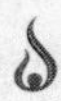

Gall Bladder Stones

Did you know that women are twice as likely as men to develop gallstones? Yes, it's true!

Excess estrogen from pregnancy, hormone replacement therapy, and birth control pills increases cholesterol levels in bile and decreases gallbladder movement, which can lead to gallstones.

Consider the case of Mrs Sodhi. Ever since her husband joined an international airline company as a pilot, her nights have been sleepless. The workload and timings for the domestic flights where her husband was previously employed were much convenient for them. But now, she doesn't get to see him for days on end.

When she visited my clinic, Mrs Sodhi told me that she had been diagnosed with gall bladder stone in 2008. She complained of bloating of the abdomen, belching, and pain in her scapular area. A disturbed sleep, anxiety, and headache were other symptoms that were diagnosed. She also had lower back pain and suffered from extreme tiredness and lethargy. On further enquiry, she told me how her husband used to travel a lot and she was finding it difficult to cope with the responsibilities. She was given homeopathic and ayurvedic medicines and her condition gradually improved over a period of 4 months.

Causes

Factors that contribute to the formation of gallstones, particularly cholesterol stones, include:

- Gender.
- Family history: Gallstones often run in families, pointing to a possible genetic link.
- Weight: Clinical study shows that being even moderately overweight increases the risk for developing gallstones. The most likely reason is that the amount of bile salts in bile is reduced, resulting in more cholesterol. Increased cholesterol reduces gallbladder emptying. Obesity is a major risk factor for gallstones, especially in women.
- Diet: A diet high in fat and cholesterol and low in fibre increases the risk of gallstones due to increased cholesterol in the bile and reduced gallbladder emptying.
- Rapid weight loss: As the body metabolizes fat during prolonged fasting and rapid weight loss—such as 'crash diets'—the liver secretes extra cholesterol into bile, which can cause gallstones. In addition, the gallbladder does not empty properly.

- Age: People older than age 60 are more likely to develop gallstones than younger people. As people age, the body tends to secrete more cholesterol into bile.
- Cholesterol-lowering drugs: Drugs that lower cholesterol levels in the blood actually increase the amount of cholesterol secreted into bile. In turn, the risk of gallstones increases.
- Diabetes: People with diabetes generally have high levels of fatty acids called triglycerides. These fatty acids may increase the risk of gallstones.

Common symptoms

- Gallstones may be asymptomatic, even for years. These gallstones are called 'silent stones' and do not require treatment.
- Symptoms commonly begin to appear once the stones reach a certain size.
- A person may experience intense pain in the upper-right side of the abdomen, accompanied by nausea and vomiting, that will last for approximately 30 minutes to several hours.
- A patient may also experience referred pain between the shoulder blades or below the right shoulder.
- Often, attacks occur after a particularly fatty meal and almost always happen at night.
- Other symptoms include abdominal bloating, intolerance of fatty foods, belching, gas, and indigestion.

Types

On the basis of their composition, gallstones can be divided into the following types:

- Cholesterol stones: Cholesterol is held in solution in bile by its association with bile acids and phospholipids. Here the liver produces bile which contains a relative excess of cholesterol.

- Pigment stones: Pigment stones are small, dark stones made of bilirubin and calcium salts that are found in bile. They are formed due to bacterial or parasitic infection in the biliary tree.
- Mixed stones: Mixed gallstones typically contain 20–80 percent cholesterol. Other common constituents are calcium carbonate, phosphate, bilirubin, and other bile pigments. Because of their calcium content, they are often radiographically visible.

When should you see a doctor?

Consult a doctor immediately if the following symptoms arise:

- Pain in the right upper abdomen, right flank or right shoulder that lasts for more than 5 hours.
- Nausea and vomiting.
- Fever—even low-grade—or chills.
- Yellowish colour of the skin or in the whites of the eyes.
- Clay-coloured stool.
- Loss of appetite.

Prevention

- Maintain a healthy weight. Sudden loss of weight and sudden gaining weight increases the risk for gallstones.
- Eat regular, balanced meals. Do not skip meals. Do eat plenty of whole grains and fibre. Have foods that contain calcium like milk products and green leafy vegetables. Limit saturated (animal) fat and foods high in cholesterol.
- Exercise regularly.

Holistic approach

A holistic approach with ayurveda, yoga, homeopathic medicines, and diet can solve this problem in a non-invasive manner. Water plays a major role in cure. Drink adequate amount of warm water.

Homeopathy

Homeopathic medicines like Chelidonium and Colocynthis can dissolve the stones. To avoid recurrence of gall stones, constitutional remedies are given. In severe condition like acute cholecystitis with severe pain, fever, and tenderness, medicines like Belladonna, Dioscorea are of important value. Homeopathy medicines are effective in alleviating pain as well as the chronic inflammation of gallbladder (cholecystitis) associated with the condition.

Naturopathy

Naturopathic treatments like abdominal pack or local mud application to abdomen, hip baths, and gastro-hepatic pack help in gall stone complaints.

Ayurveda

Numerous herbs known as Cholagogues and Choleretics have been found useful in preventing gallstones in traditional ayurvedic medicine. Cholagogues are herbs that stimulate the gallbladder to contract, while Choleretics stimulate the liver to secrete more bile. Both these actions could help reduce the risk of developing gallstones. Turmeric, citrus fruits, dried ginger, black pepper, long pepper, and hing fall under these categories. Apatarpana (fasting), langhana (light diet) and virechana (mild purgation) are some of the therapeutic procedures that are usually advised as a part of the treatment.

Yoga

Chandra Nadi Pranayama and relaxation techniques are also good for gall bladder complaints in addition to asanas like Vakrasana, Baradwajasana, Pawanmuktasana, Ardha Matsyendrasana, and Salabhasana.

Kitchen cures

- Drink 8–10 glasses of water in a day to maintain the water content of bile.
- Vitamin C is needed to convert cholesterol to bile acids. In theory, such a conversion should reduce gallstone risks. So, consume Vitamin-C rich fruits such as aamla and citrus fruits.
- Apply castor oil pack over the gallbladder area. Take a cup of castor oil, and soak a flannel cloth in it. Place the saturated cloth over the gallbladder area, and cover with plastic. Over the plastic, apply a heating pad, and leave it on for half an hour. Initially, do this once a day, every day for a month. Continue the treatment thrice a week, increasing use of the packs during an acute condition.

DR MATHAI'S TIPS

- Do not overeat.
- Avoid packaged food and food with preservatives.
- Exercise daily.
- Maintain a healthy lifestyle.
- Include lot of fruits in your daily diet.

Seven Qualities Of A Holistic Doctor

1. He takes more time with you

The holistic doctor will ask you about your family, your social life, your emotional life and listen carefully to your answers, understand your lifestyle, and eating habits. Many diseases originate after an emotional trauma, unhappy marriage or job, bad eating habits, and lifestyles.

2. He considers the mind-body connection

Instead of dismissing complaints as all in your head, he sees the mind as a truly powerful organ that can cause both healing and disease. He understands the role that meditation, psychological counselling and spirituality can play in the healing process.

3. He helps you harness your body's self-healing power

He understands that he is not the healer—your body and mind is. You hold that power. He advises you and helps you to enhance your self-healing power.

4. He gives you the choice of treatment options

He tells you about the many possibilities available, rather than assume there's only one right way. He offers you his recommendations but respects and supports your choices should the two of you differ. He has an open mind, being aware about the different systems of medicine, modalities, and therapies can help in healing a person so he can direct you towards the right direction based on his knowledge.

5. He will reassure you about the positive aspects to your condition

Instead of telling you about the statistics associated with your diagnosis, your doctor will assume that the pace and likelihood of your recovery will be as individual as you are, even if the statistics say that only one person in a thousand will recover, there is no reason to believe that the patient might not be you.

6. He lives the healthy lifestyle he preaches

Instead of a medical training and practice system that requires doctors to forgo sleep, exercise, proper nutrition, and a spiritual life, the holistic doctor will eat wisely and well, exercise for both health and joy, and have time to meditate and think and do the best for the patient.

7. He is honest

A holistic doctor is honest about what he can do and what he cannot. He explains the benefits and limitations of different systems of medicine to the patient and advises the best way possible and the right combination of treatments the person should take. He is willing to refer you to another doctor or system.

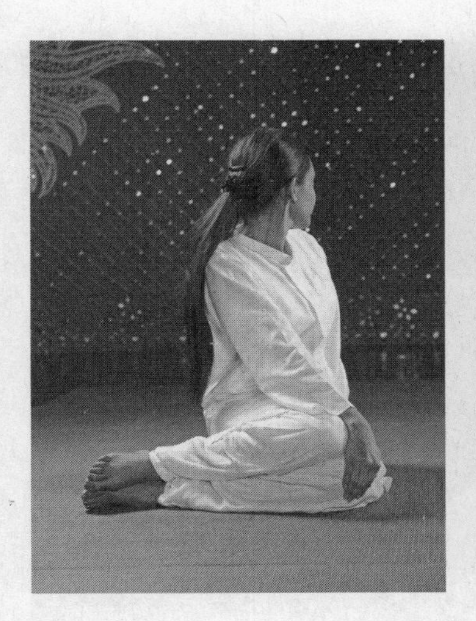

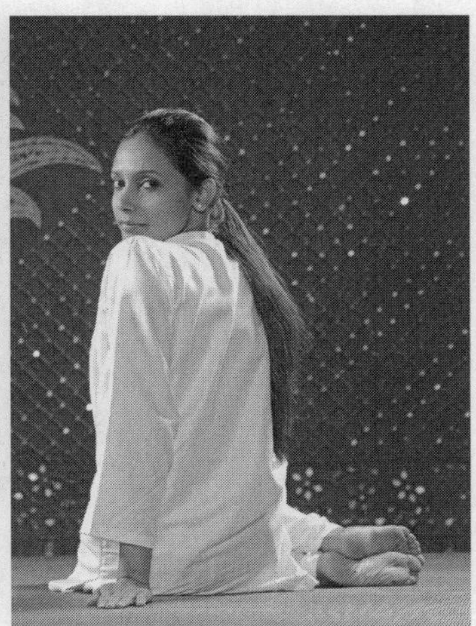

Bharadvajasana

- Sit with the legs stretched.
- Bend the legs at the knees, such that the right knee is on top of the left and right ankle on top of the left ankle.
- Place the right hand on the left knee.
- Place the left hand behind the spine, as close as possible, to support and be able to hold the spine straight.
- With an exhalation turn the head backwards and look to the back.
- You will feel the stretch in the shoulders, neck, and hips.
- Mild compression is felt in the lower abdomen and pelvis.
- With inhalation, turn the head to the front.
- Release the right hand, then the left.
- Straighten the right leg and release the left.
- Now repeat it on the other side.

Benefits

Strengthens the pelvic muscles • Tones the uterus and the reproductive system

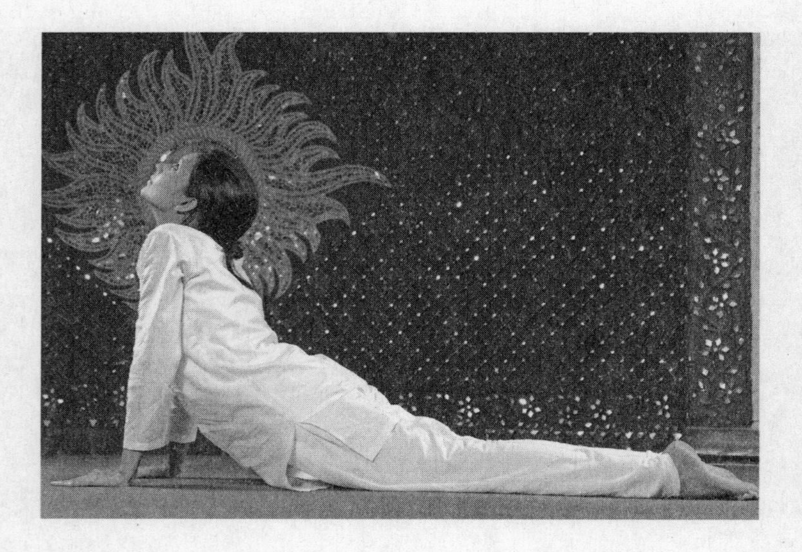

Bhujangasana (cobra pose)

- Lie on the abdomen with legs together, palms placed by the side of the chest facing down.
- Let the chin touch the ground. With an inhalation, start raising the chin, chest and abdomen up to the navel up.
- Breathe normally and feel the compression in the mid back region.
- Breathe normally and hold it comfortably.
- With an exhalation, slowly lower the body first placing the chest and then chin on the ground.
- Release the hands, keep the legs apart, and relax.

Benefits

Bhujangasana strengthens the shoulders and mid back region

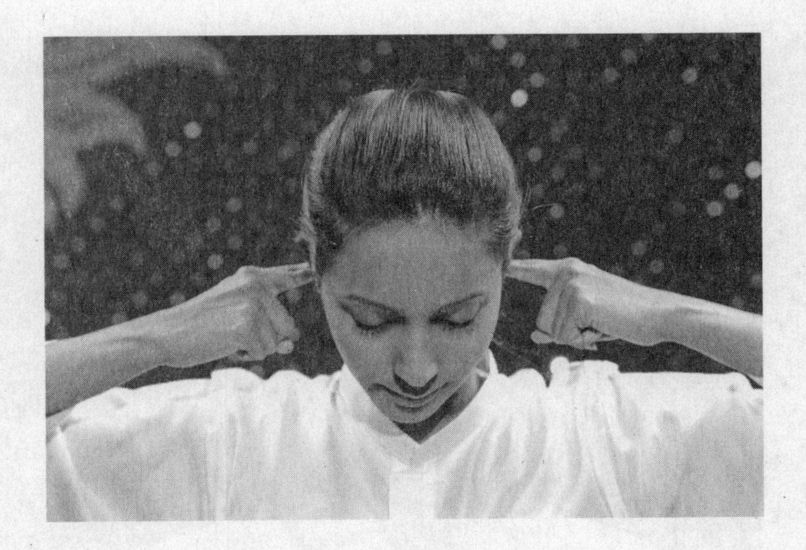

Bhramari Pranayama

Brahmari means the sound made by the male bee to attract the female bee. This pranayama is called so, because we try and imitate the same sound. During the practice, there are sound vibrations created and it resonates in the brain. It is proven that these vibrations cause the multiplication of grey cells in the brain. This improves the concentration, memory, and intelligence.

Inhale through the nostrils. Plug the ears with a convenient finger. As you exhale, lower the head to touch the chin to the notch in the throat and all the while making a humming sound in the throat. With an inhalation, straighten the head and repeat the above with an exhalation.

Practice it for 9-27 rounds.

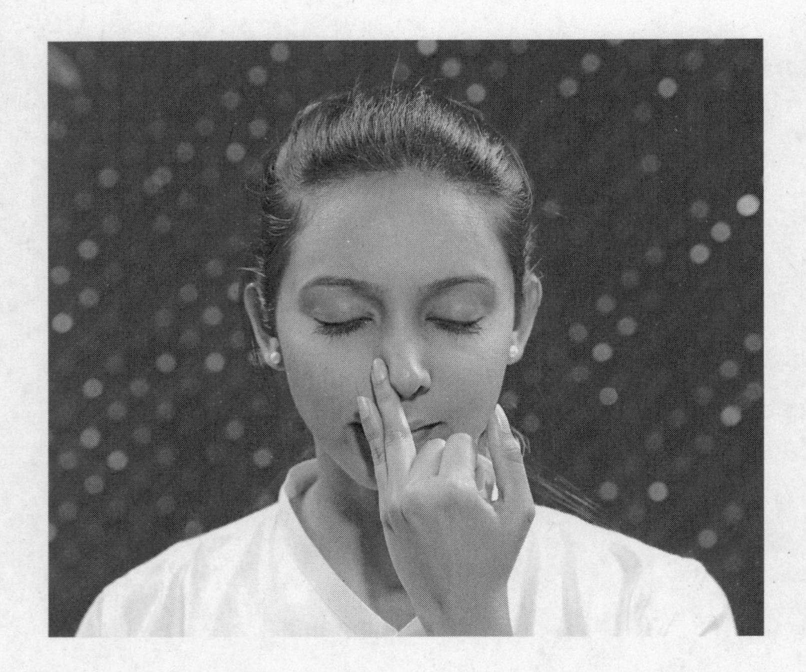

Chandra Nadi Pranayama

Inhale and exhale only through the left nostril, by entirely closing the right.

This can be practiced only if there are no conflicting symptoms.

Benefits

Good in cases of hypertension, irritability, excessive hunger and hyperacidity, and anxiety

CHAPTER THREE

Circulatory System

THE CIRCULATORY SYSTEM COMPRISES OF THE HEART AND the blood vessels like the arteries, veins, and capillaries. The function of the circulatory system is to ensure proper supply of oxygenated blood to the cells, tissues, and organs. The blood vessels carry the impure blood from the whole body, get it oxygenated and purified with the help of the lungs, and through the heart, taking it back to the organs and systems in the body. The circulatory system also include the lymphatics, which carry the toxins for elimination and the lymph to the organs which is an integral part of the body's defence mechanism.

But there are many diseases that plague the circulatory system. Let's take a look at the most potent ones.

Cholestrol

If you think you're only one in a few suffering from cholesterol, think again! A 2011 survey conducted by a chain of diagnostic clinics ahead of the World Heart Day revealed that men between 25 and 45 years in Ahmedabad had alarmingly high cholesterol and triglyceride levels, which are one of the key risk factors for heart disease. Of these, 25 percent men were found to be suffering from high or abnormal levels of cholesterol and triglyceride in their blood stream. This prevalence is alarming as a study conducted by the South Asian Health Centre among Asian Indian men which showed that half of all heart attacks in this population occur under the age of 50 years, and 25 percent under the age of 40.

In fact, local doctors have been reporting a higher trend of heart attacks in young people, especially men in their 20s, 30s, and 40s.

Hyperlipidemia (high cholesterol) occurs due to various factors. The contributing factors could be either genetic or acquired. It could be a consequence of unhealthy eating and lifestyle, metabolic disorders, or thyroid malfunction. The raised lipids cause a major threat to the circulatory system. It could affect the heart, brain, and other vital organs.

A cholesterol level of over 200 mg/dl, Triglycerides over 100 mg/dl, LDL (Low density lipoprotein) of more than 70 mg/dl, and HDL (High density lipoprotein) below 30 mg/dl are all considered to be risky and are collectively termed as Hyperlipidemia.

Women around menopausal age tend to develop hyperlipidemia. Generally the metabolism gets sluggish with menopause due to hormonal changes. The fat metabolism in particular gets affected. This is the time women tend to get inactive, which contributes to the condition as well. As a result dyslipidemia sets in. Sometimes it also accompanies hypothyroidism and diabetes.

It could be easily controlled to a large extent through right eating and proper exercises, if the contributing factor is not major.

Prevention

- Eating non-spicy, low-fat food, including green leaves,

coloured vegetables and fruits in the diet all help reduce the cholesterol.

- Intake of adequate water.
- Taking 3-4 raw garlic cloves on empty stomach reduces the triglycerides.
- Avoid red meat, shell fish and crustaceans, egg yolk and cashew nuts. Including omega-3 fatty acids through seeds and nuts such as alfalfa, sunflower seeds, pumpkin seeds, flaxseeds and nuts like almonds, walnuts, and pistachios protect the heart and nervous system.
- Avoiding alcohol helps a lot in controlling lipids. Regular exercise is a must to reduce the fat and also to strengthen the arteries and establish proper circulation. Regular walking and yoga including asana, pranayamas, and meditation help to control the cholesterol.

Holistic approach

Holistically we look at improving and setting right the metabolism through liver detoxification, and balancing the hormonal secretions which is done through various therapies from different systems of medicine and internal medications. Lifestyle modifications are also advised.

Treatments like liver pack, abdomen compress, hip baths and mud packs help to control the cholesterol. Diet is an integral part of naturopathy and going on raw diet, fruits, and juices help a lot in reducing the cholesterol.

Homeopathy

Aurum met, Cholestrinum, and constitutional powders are prescribed.

Ayurveda

Internal medications containing garlic, turmeric, piper longum (pippali), piper nigrum (pepper) and embelica officinalis (amla) are prescribed to control the cholesterol.

Blood Pressure

If recent surveys are anything to go by, more than a third of young people suffer from high blood pressure. This may seem shocking to many considering the fact that it is commonly believed that blood pressure is a problem one encounters in old age.

Causes

Main causes are hereditary, stress, sedentary lifestyles, obesity, smoking, and poor eating habits.

Common symptoms

Most of the times, it is symptomless, though sometimes palpitations, occipital headache, giddiness, nausea, or chest pain can be felt.

Types

Blood pressure could be termed as high or low based on various factors like age, sex, time of the day, genetics, and demography. Though 120/80 mm hg is considered as normal blood pressure, it cannot be generalized.

A sustained diastolic pressure (the lower gradient) greater than 90 mm hg and a sustained systolic pressure (upper gradient) in excess of 140 mm hg is generally diagnosed as hypertension. Likewise, a pressure less than 70 mm hg diastolic and 100 mm hg systolic is considered as low blood pressure.

Hypertension or high blood pressure is a common health problem. It is an important risk factor in both coronary heart disease and cerebrovascular accidents. Some of the complications of hypertension are angina pectoris and other cardiac complaints, stroke, and paralysis.

Holistic approach

Homeopathy

Internal medications to calm the mind and strengthen the heart are given which include Natrum Muraticum 200, Aurum Met, Rowalfia Q, and Belladona.

Naturopathy

Hydrotherapic treatments like wet compresses, chest compresses, mud bath, spinal bath, and ice application to the neck and spine are helpful.

Ayurveda

Ayurvedic treatments mainly aim at de-stressing and strengthening the heart and the nervous systems.

The treatments include Sirodhara and Thalam to strengthen the nervous system and to de-stress.

Abhyanga, Padabhyanga, Choorna Swedam etc. are done to improve the circulation and to strengthen the blood vessels. Special treatments are done to improve the heart function.

Internal medications are given to strengthen the heart and nervous system and to de-stress. They are combinations containing herbs such as Raulfia Serpentine, Garlic, Phylanthrum Niruri (Bhoomiamlaki), Stevia, Arjuna (Terminalia Arjuna) and Patola (Trichosanthes Diodica).

Yoga

Asanas, pranayamas, deep relaxation technique, yoga nidra, and deep breathing help to balance the Prana, improve the heart and lungs, and to relax and strengthen the nervous system.

Acupressure and Reflexology
Relieves excessive tension and trapped nerves while strengthening internal organs.

Acupuncture
Improves sleep and relaxes the mind.

Diet
Nutritional evaluation needs to be done first and then dietary advice is given to strengthen the heart and blood vessels. Ash gourd juice, beetroot soup, barley water, tender coconut water, plantain stem juice, and juice of drumstick leaves are all seen to reduce the blood pressure.

Palpitations

Palpitations are something most of us experience on an everyday basis. They occur due to some of the valvular diseases of the heart, due to stress, anxiety, and panic or as a result of hormonal changes which occur at menopause. We need to understand the reason behind the attacks. The treatments would be administered accordingly.

Yoga, pranayamas, and meditation help a lot in controlling the palpitations as it checks the anxiety and stress levels. It also improves the circulation and strengthens the muscles and nerves which includes the heart too and hence, reduces palpitations.

Holistic Approach

Homeopathy

Aconite 30, Digitalis 30, Cactus 30, and Gelsemium 200 are all seen to reduce palpitations.

Naturopathy

Chest packs and spinal bath are seen to control palpitations.

Ayurveda

Treatments to strengthen the muscles and nerves, to improve circulation, and to de-stress are given which include Sirodhara, Abhyanga, Hrid Vasti, and Thalam. Internal medications to strengthen the heart and the nervous system are prescribed too. These include herbs such as Arjuna, Rauwolfia, Phylanthus Niruri (Bhoomiamlaki), and Borhevia Diffusa (Punarnava).

DIETS FOR VARIOUS CONDITIONS

	CONDITION	RECOMMENDED DIET
1	Hypothyroidism	Natural foods, whole grains, lots of fruits and vegetables, good supply of seafood and other lean protein. Foods such as tuna, brown rice, Brazil nuts, and salmon can provide the selenium. Fish, lentils, and low-fat milk as these are rich in tyrosine, green tea, fibre foods, coconut oil, water, and other iodine-rich foods. To be excluded: Soya and its products, cabbage, cauliflower, broccoli, brussels sprouts.
2	Diabetes	1. Bread and flour products: Rye bread, wheat protein, protein-bran. 2. Meat and poultry: Lean beef, veal, lamb, pork and meat edged, rabbit, chicken minced and pieces, boiled and steamed fried. Lean ham, beef sausages. 3. Fish: Low-fat baked, boiled and occasionally in the form of fried; limited soaked herring, canned in tomato sauce.

Contd...

	CONDITION	RECOMMENDED DIET
		Eggs: 1 whole egg or 2 egg whites recommended. 5. Dairy products: Milk, yogurt, kefir, cottage cheese or low-fat, bold, cheese. To be excluded: Sweet curd cheese, cream. 6. Fats: Butter and vegetable oil. To be excluded: Meat and cooking oils. 7. Cereals, pasta, and beans: Porridge from barley, buckwheat, millet, oats, peas should be limited and subject to rules of carbohydrates. To be excluded: Semolina, rice, pasta. 8. Vegetables: Cabbage, lettuce, pumpkin, squash, cucumbers, tomatoes, eggplants. To be excluded: Marinated and pickled products. 9. Soups: Lean meat, fish, mushrooms broth, with potatoes, vegetables, soup, cabbage, beetroot, (meat and vegetables). 10. Fruits, desserts, and sweets: Sweet-sour fruit and berries in any form. To be excluded: Grapes, raisins, dates, figs, bananas, sugar, honey, jam, candy, ice cream. 11. Drinks: Tea, coffee, cocoa and milk, no sugar, unsweetened juices of fresh fruits and berries, and tomato juice. To be excluded: Sweet fruit and berry juices (grape, etc.), sweet brew carbonated drinks with sugar.
3	Hypertension	Water soluble gel-forming fibres such as oat bran, apple pectin, psyllium seeds, and guar gum. Take 1–3 tablespoons of herbal bulking formula such as ginger root powder, fenugreek seed powder, and fennel seed powder. A diet that is rich in high potassium foods (vegetables and fruits) bananas, oranges, apricots, avocado, strawberries, potatoes, tomatoes,

Contd...

	CONDITION	RECOMMENDED DIET
		cucumber, cabbage, cauliflower, bell pepper, eggplant, squash, sprouts, turmeric, parsley, spinach, broccoli, tuna. Essential fatty acids—Celery, garlic, onion, and carrots.
4	Arthritis	1. Pineapple: Rheumatoid arthritis causes inflammation around the point where joints connects each other. Pineapples contain Bromelain that acts as an agent to reduce the production of prostaglandins which is a major reason for inflammation around joints. 2. Ginger: Have some ginger with carrot juice and apple. It will help in curing arthritis; it acts exactly like antibiotics to lower inflammation. 3. Indian gooseberry: Amla helps in reducing inflammation around joints and they also heal wear and tear of joints. (Note: Eat only fresh Indian gooseberry or Amla and its juice, not preservatives.) 4. Garlic: It has anti-inflammatory properties that helps in treating infections in the body caused due to arthritis. 5. Ground nut: It helps in the prevention of malnutrition andvascular complications by maintaining the level of synovial fluid or liquid gel around joints. 6. Basil tea: It is the right substitute for tea and coffee and it also lowers inflammation arthritis pain. 7. Grapefruit: It lowers the level of blood sugar and carbohydrates which are a major cause for arthritis. 8. Lemon tea: Has anti-inflammatory properties. 9. Carrots: Arthritis is caused mostly because of indigestion and carrots are the best resource for proper digestion and to lower inflammation internally.

Contd...

	CONDITION	RECOMMENDED DIET
		10. Neem: Swallow young leaves of neem directly. They not only lower inflammation but are also a great cure for arthritis. 11. Pomegranates: This fruit gives inner strength to fight infections and is a powerful tool to cure arthritis.
5	Bone Health	1. Milk: Our bones need calcium to stay healthy and strong. Milk is one of the richest sources of calcium. 2. Yogurt and cheese: Dairy products like yogurt and cheese are the next best foods for healthy bones. 3. Green leafy vegetables: Many vegetables like Chinese cabbage and broccoli are great sources of calcium as well as proteins required for healthy and flexible bones. 4. Soy foods: recent studies have shown that calcium isn't the only nutrient needed for strong bones. Plant-based chemicals called Isoflavones are also needed to strengthen bone density. 5. Nuts and seeds: Nuts like almonds, pistachios, and seeds like sunflower seeds, seaweeds are very rich in calcium content as well as minerals such as iron, boron, selenium, phosphorus, and magnesium.
6	Constipation	1. Dark leafy greens such as spinach, broccoli and cauliflower, eggplant, celery, green peas, tomatoes. 2. Dried peas and beans such as kidney beans, lima beans, black-eyed beans, chick peas and lentils. 3. Dried fruits such as apricots, dates, prunes and raisins. 4. Berries and fruits such as blackberries, blueberries, raspberries and strawberries, oranges, apples with skin, avocado, kiwi, mango and pear.

Contd...

	CONDITION	RECOMMENDED DIET
		5. Whole grains such as barley, popcorn, corn and brown rice. 6. Cooked cereal such as red river and oat bran, whole grain breads andbuns.
7	Hair Health	1. Salmon: Loaded with omega-3 fatty acids, this high-quality protein source is also filled with Vitamin B-12 and iron. Essential omega-3 fatty acids are needed to support scalp health, A deficiency can result in a dry scalp and thus hair, giving it a dull look. Include one or two tablespoons of ground flaxseed in your daily diet for some plant-based omega-3 fats. 2. Dark green vegetables: Spinach, like broccoli and Swiss chard, is an excellent source of Vitamins A and C, which your body needs to produce sebum. The oily substance secreted by your hair follicles is the body's natural hair conditioner. Dark green vegetables also provide iron and calcium. 3. Beans: Beans like kidney beans and lentils should be an important part of your haircare diet. Not only do they provide plentiful protein to promote hair growth, but ample iron, zinc, and biotin. While rare, biotin deficiencies can result in brittle hair. 4. Nuts: Brazil nuts are one of nature's best sources of selenium, an important mineral for the health of your scalp. Walnuts contain alpha-linolenic acid, an omega-3 fatty acid that may help condition your hair. They are also a terrific source of zinc, as are cashews, pecans, and almonds. A zinc deficiency can lead to hair shedding, so make sure nuts are a regular on your healthy hair menu. 5. Poultry: Chickens and turkeys may have feathers, but the high-quality protein they provide will help give you the healthy hair you crave. Without adequate protein or with

Contd...

	CONDITION	RECOMMENDED DIET
		low-quality protein, one can experience weak brittle hair, while a profound protein deficiency can result in loss of hair colour. 6. Eggs: When it comes to healthy hair, it doesn't matter whether you like your eggs scrambled, fried, or over easy. However eggs are one of the best protein sources you can find. They also contain biotin and Vitamin B-12, which are important beauty nutrients. 7. Whole grains: Sink your teeth into hearty whole grains, including wholewheat bread and fortified whole-grain breakfast cereals, for a hair-healthy dose of zinc, iron, and B vitamins. 8. Oysters: Oysters may be better known for their reputation as an aphrodisiac, but they can also lead to healthy hair. 9. Low-fat dairy products: Low-fat dairy products like skim milk and yogurt are great sources of calcium, an important mineral for hair growth. They also contain whey and casein, two high-quality protein sources. 10. Carrots: Carrots are an excellent source of Vitamin A, which promotes a healthy scalp along with good vision. Since a healthy scalp is essential for a shiny, well-conditioned head of hair, you'd be wise to include carrots in your diet as snacks or toppings on your salad.
8	Skin Health	1. Green tea: Green tea is rich in antioxidants that reduce inflammation and protect cell membranes. It has been proven to reduce the damage of sunburns and overexposure to ultraviolet light, which in turn reduces the risk of skin cancer. Green tea is also high in polyphenols—compounds that eliminate cancer-causing free radicals.

Contd...

	CONDITION	RECOMMENDED DIET
		2. Salmon: Along with other fatty fish, walnuts and flaxseed, Salmon is high in healthy fatty acids that are key for achieving healthy skin. Essential fatty acids such as omega-3s help keep cell membranes healthy by keeping out harmful substances as well as allowing nutrients to enter cells and exit with waste products. Omega-3s also reduce the body's production of inflammatory agents that can damage the skin. Increasing consumption of omega-3 fatty acid-rich foods such as salmon will help keep the skin supple and youthful. 3. Blueberries: Blueberries are considered by many experts to be the food source for highest levels of antioxidants, which target free radicals that can wreak havoc on skin cells. 4. Carrots: Carrots are an excellent source of Vitamin A, which is a required nutrient for healthy skin. They also contain high levels of antioxidants, which prevent free radical damage of skin cells. Vitamin A is required for developing and maintaining skin cells, and a deficiency of the vitamin can cause dry skin. 5. Water: Drinking plenty of water—at least your individual minimum intake—will help keep your skin young and healthy-looking. Water in caffeinated or sugary beverages does not count; water intake must be from pure, clean water, which rejuvenates skin cells. Water both hydrates cells and helps them move toxins out and nutrients in. When the body is properly hydrated, it sweats more efficiently, which helps keep the skin clean and clear.
9	Obesity	1. Juices of lemon, grapefruit, orange, pineapple, strawberries, watermelon. 2. Vegetables like cabbage and gourds (ash and bottle), broccoli, cabbage, carrots,

Contd...

	CONDITION	RECOMMENDED DIET
		cauliflower, celery, cucumbers green beans, kale, lettuce, onions, radishes, spinach, turnips, lentils, tofu, sesame seeds, beans. Incorporate high-fibre and unrefined complex carbohydrates, such as whole grains because the body is less successful digesting these and feels full sooner than with refined carbohydrates, such as sugar and white flour. 3. Eat raw or lightly cooked vegetables. 4. Consume protein with low amounts of saturated fat, including dry peas and beans. 5. Non vegetarian foods like skinless turkey, chicken breast, whitefish.
10	Headaches/ Migraine	Anti-inflammatory Diet to include: 1. Vitamin D—Vit D deficiency is common, even with adequate sun exposure. 2. Low carbs—Starch is hyperglycemic and grain gluten intolerance is very common. 3. Vegetable oils—Only olive oil is safe (Trans fats are dangerous), butter is better. 4. Fish oil—Omega-3 oils can reduce chronic inflammation. 5. Eliminate all sources of High fructose corn syrup. 6. Saturated Fats—safer than polyunsaturated fats but are amajor source of calories. The best advice is to simply to eat a well balanced diet with plenty of fresh, non-processed foods. That includes a variety of grains, fruits and vegetables. Peppermint, cayenne pepper, ginger, fish and fish oil, foods rich in calcium (such as spinach, broccoli and kale) and foods rich in magnesium such as spinach oatmeal, wheat, garlic are healthy.

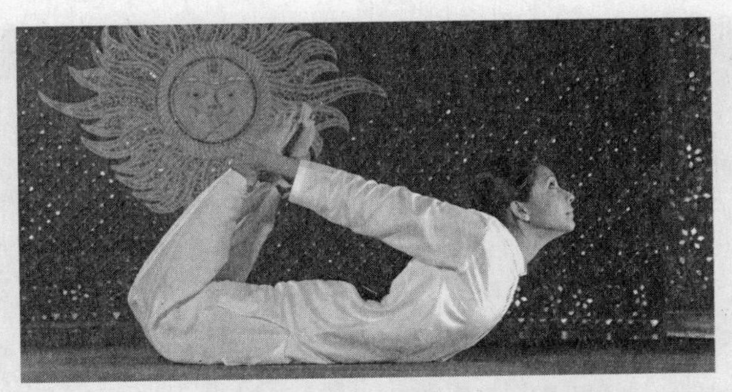

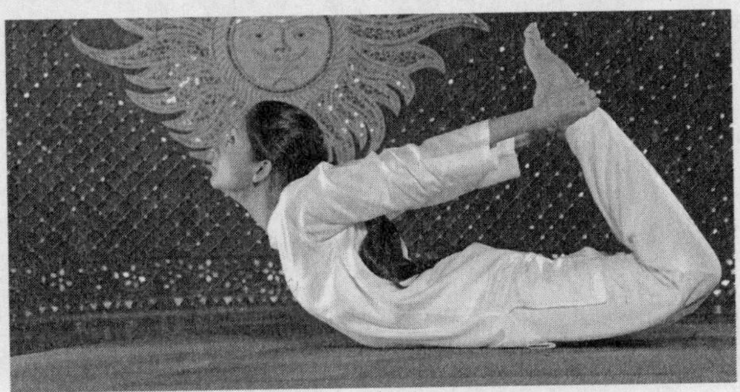

Dhanurasana

- Lie on your abdomen, legs together, chin touching the ground and hands placed by the sides of the chest
- Bend the legs at the knees, bringing the feet closer to the buttocks.
- Hold the ankles with the respective hands (you could also hold the toes, if that's comfortable).
- With an inhalation, simultaneously lift up the chin, chest and abdomen and the thighs, to give the body a shape of a bow.
- Hold this posture with normal breathing.
- With an exhalation, slowly place the abdomen, thighs, chest and chin back on the floor.
- Release the legs and hands.

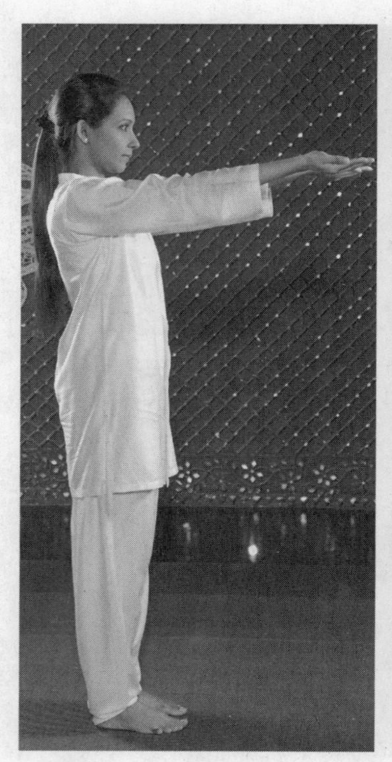

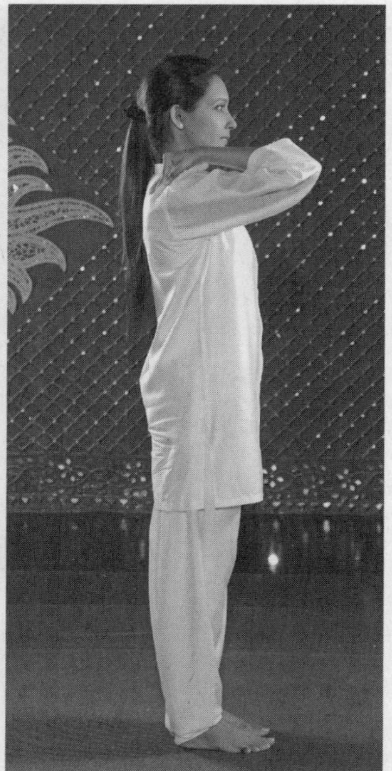

Elbow Movements

- Stretch the arms in front of your body.
- With inhalation flex the elbow and with exhalation extend it.
- Apart from the elbows, the changes are felt in the biceps and triceps.

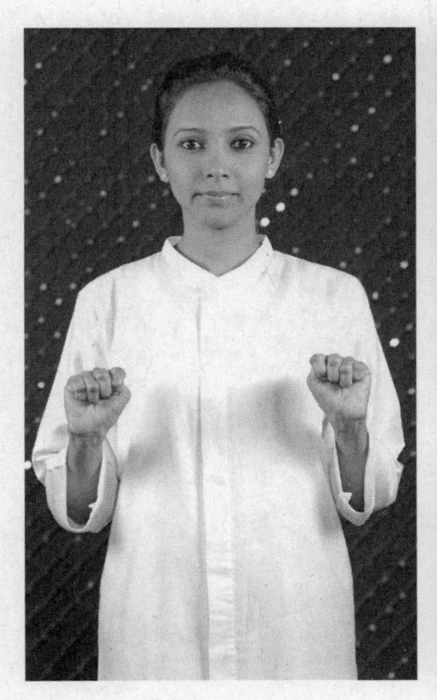

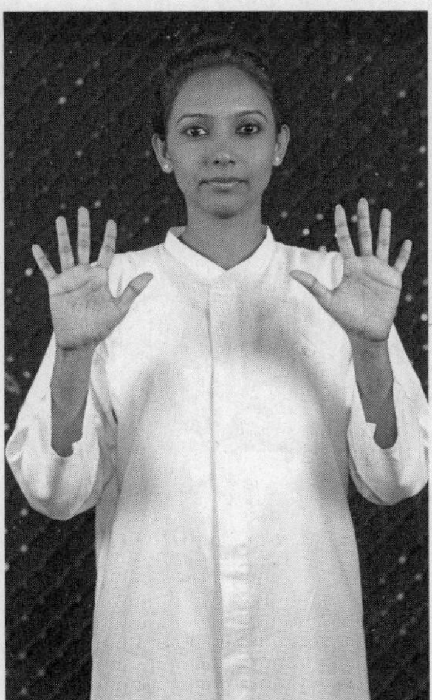

Finger Movements

- Make a tight fist as you inhale and release them as you exhale.
- Feel the tension from the whole upper half of the body getting relieved.

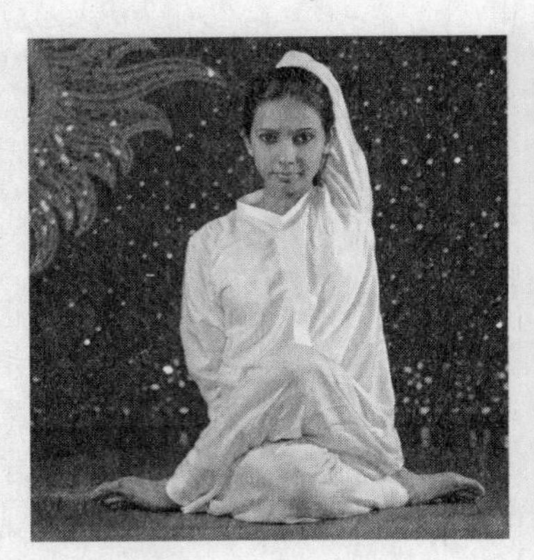

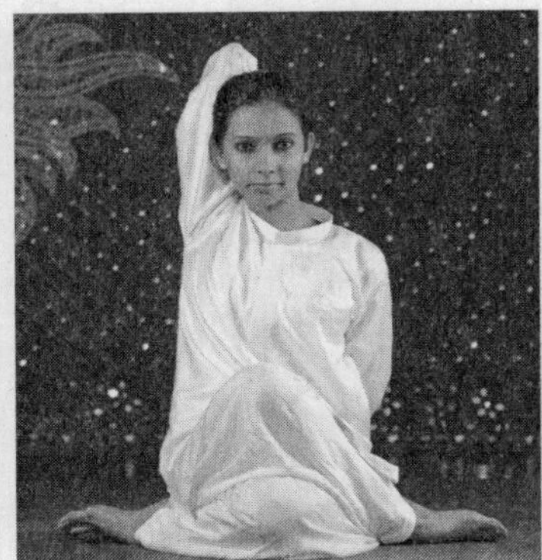

Gomukhasana (cow's face pose)

- Sit straight with the legs extended.
- Bend the right leg and place it beneath the left thigh.
- Now cross the left leg on top of the right, such that the left knee is placed on the right knee.
- With an inhalation, take the left hand from above the shoulder and right hand from below to join the fingers, if possible. If not, hold where ever you can comfortably.
- Make sure, the neck is held straight.
- Feel the stretch in the entire spine, shoulders, hips, and thighs.
- This asana improves the posture, improves digestive function, and relieves the neck and back stiffness.
- With an exhalation, first release the left hand and then the right.
- Release the left leg and then the right.
- Relax with the legs stretched.
- Now start doing it on the other side, by placing the left leg beneath the right leg and right knee on top of the left.
- Take the right hand up and left hand from below with an inhalation.
- Hold the posture comfortably with normal breathing.
- Release the hands and then the legs.
- Relax the whole body.

CHAPTER FOUR

Cancers

Breast Cancer

BREAST CANCER IS A CANCER THAT STARTS IN THE TISSUES of the breast. Breasts start to develop with puberty. The size and shape of the breasts differ according to individual body structure and heredity. Breast development is part of the preparation of a woman's body for sexual life, reproduction, and lactation.

Self examination of breasts

Congenitally, there could be certain problems with the breasts like inverted nipples and hairy breasts. These could be corrected through proper medical advice and through simple home remedies like regular massages.

Generally with periods, certain symptoms like heaviness of the breasts, tenderness etc. can occur. At this time, on palpation, small cysts could be found too. They may or may not be painful. They tend to disappear with periods. This generally happens with people who have fibrous breasts.

Apart from and irrespective of periods, if the breasts are tender, cystic, one needs to see a gynaecologist.

Routine breast examination helps early diagnosis of malignant conditions.

One could follow the steps below:

Step 1: Begin by looking at your breasts in the mirror with your shoulders straight and your arms on your hips.

Here's what you should look for:

- Breasts that are their usual size, shape, and colour.
- Breasts that are evenly shaped without visible distortion or swelling.

If you see any of the following changes, bring them to your doctor's attention:

- Dimpling, puckering, or bulging of the skin.
- A nipple that has changed position or an inverted nipple (pushed inward instead of sticking out).
- Redness, soreness, rash, or swelling.

Step 2: Now, raise your arms and look for the same changes.

Step 3: While you're at the mirror, look for any signs of fluid coming out of one or both nipples (this could be a watery, milky, or yellow fluid or blood).

Step 4: Next, feel your breasts while lying down, using your right hand to feel your left breast and then your left hand to feel your right breast. Use a firm, smooth touch with the first few finger pads of your hand, keeping the fingers flat and together. Use a circular motion, about the size of a quarter.

Cover the entire breast from top to bottom, side to side—from your collarbone to the top of your abdomen, and from your armpit to your cleavage.

Follow a pattern to be sure that you cover the whole breast.

You can begin at the nipple, moving in larger and larger circles until you reach the outer edge of the breast. You can also move your fingers up and down vertically, in rows, as if you were mowing a lawn. This up-and-down approach seems to work best for most women. Be sure to feel all the tissue from the front to the back of your breasts: for the skin and tissue just beneath, use light pressure; use medium pressure for tissue in the middle of your breasts; use firm pressure for the deep tissue in the back. When you've reached the deep tissue, you should be able to feel down to your ribcage.

Step 5: Finally, feel your breasts while you are standing or sitting. Many women find that the easiest way to feel their breasts is when their skin is wet and slippery, so they like to do this in the shower. Cover your entire breast, using the same hand movements described in Step 4.

After the examination, if any doubt arises, do not hesitate to meet the gynaecologist and under go further tests such as ultrasound, mammography etc.

Causes and risk factors

Risk factors you cannot change include:

- Age and gender—Your risk of developing breast cancer increases as you get older. Most advanced breast cancer cases are found in women over age 50. Women are 100 times more likely to get breast cancer than men.
- Family history of breast cancer—You may also have a higher risk for breast cancer if you have a close relative who has had breast, uterine, ovarian, or colon cancer. About 20–30 percent of women with breast cancer have a family history of the disease.
- Genes—Some people have genes that make them more likely to develop breast cancer.

- Menstrual cycle—Women who got their periods early (before age 12) or went through menopause late (after age 55) have an increased risk for breast cancer.

Other risk factors include:

- Alcohol use—Drinking more than 1–2 glasses of alcohol a day may increase your risk for breast cancer.
- Childbirth—Women who have never had children or who had them only after age 30 have an increased risk for breast cancer. Being pregnant more than once or becoming pregnant at an early age reduces your risk of breast cancer.
- Hormone replacement therapy (HRT)—You have a higher risk for breast cancer if you have received hormone replacement therapy with estrogen for several years or more.

Common symptoms

Early breast cancer usually does not cause symptoms. This is why regular breast exams are important. As the cancer grows, symptoms may include:

- Breast lump or lump in the armpit that is hard, has uneven edges, and usually does not hurt.
- Change in the size, shape, or feel of the breast or nipple—for example, you may have redness, dimpling, or puckering that looks like the skin of an orange.
- Fluid coming from the nipple—may be bloody, clear to yellow, green, and looks like pus.

Symptoms of advanced breast cancer may include:

- Bone pain.
- Breast pain or discomfort.
- Skin ulcers.
- Swelling of one arm (next to the breast with cancer).
- Weight loss.

Types

There are two main types of breast cancer:

- ❖ Ductal carcinoma starts in the tubes (ducts) that move milk from the breast to the nipple. Most breast cancers are of this type.
- ❖ Lobular carcinoma starts in the parts of the breast, called lobules, that produce milk.

In rare cases, breast cancer can start in other areas of the breast.

Breast cancer may be invasive or noninvasive. Invasive means it has spread from the milk duct or lobule to other tissues in the breast. Noninvasive means it has not yet invaded other breast tissues. Noninvasive breast cancer is called 'in situ'.

When should one see a doctor?

When some change is noticed in the shape of the breast, or if the nipple turns inverted, or if any lumps are found, or if orange peel-like appearance occurs, or if any discharge is noticed from the nipples, immediately visit the doctor.

Signs and tests

MRI, PET scans, CT scans, mammography, and cancer markers.

Prevention

Self-examination of the breast regularly, and being vigilant of any changes is critical. After the age of 40 years, regular mammography should be done. This should be started earlier if one has a strong family history.

Complications

One may experience side effects or complications from cancer treatments. For example, radiation therapy may cause temporary swelling of the breast (Lymphedema), and aches and pains around the area.

Lymphedema may start 6–8 weeks after surgery or after radiation treatment for cancer.

It can also start very slowly after your cancer treatment is over. You may not notice symptoms until 18–24 months after treatment. Sometimes it can take years to develop.

Holistic approach

The holistic approach in cancer treatment focuses on providing integrative medicines along with western medicine including chemotherapy, surgery, and radiation. Modern cancer treatment is developed to such and extent that early diagnosis and specific target treatments and highly sophisticated tumour markers are identified. In our experience of treating different stages of cancer, it is always better for the patient and the disease to have an integrated approach. Lifestyle management, diet, emotional and psychological support, and spirituality are equally important for cancer management. For a very advanced cancer, homeopathic and ayurvedic treatments can be very effective to reduce the side effects of radiation and chemotherapy and boost the immune system, in turn strengthening the patients' ability to fight cancer.

In the early stages of cancer, integrated medicine is very effective along with western medicine. For the post-cancer treatment, it is very important to do homeopathic and ayurvedic treatments to change the body constitution to prevent the possibility of future recurrence.

Any disease, including cancer, arises or becomes active in favourable conditions. These favourable conditions are lowered immunity and physical or mental stress. Though one has a predisposition to certain diseases, they lie dormant if the condition does not favour. One's lifestyle contributes to making the situation favourable through accumulation of toxins. These toxins could either be physical or mental.

Through holistic approach, we can detoxify the system with

the help of integrated medical approach and maintain a healthy lifestyle through proper dietary guidelines, exercise, and yoga.

Homeopathy

Bryonia is a good remedy for breast tenderness and hardness of breast. Phytolacca, Conium, and Silicea can be used for lumps in breasts. Any abscess in the breast can be treated with Phytolacca, Silicea, and Merc Sol. These medicines can be taken in consultation with a homeopathic doctor.

Since it's a surgical case followed by chemo/radiotherapy, there are no holistic solutions other than the preventive aspects and dietary changes. Treatments involved are mainly for detoxification following the conventional intervention and to boost the immunity.

This would include treatments from all disciplines and internal medications.

Diet

- Choose foods and portion sizes that promote a healthy weight.
- Choose whole grains instead of refined grain products.
- Eat 5 or more servings of fruits and vegetables each day.
- Limit processed food and red meat in the diet.
- Limit alcohol consumption to one drink per day (women who are at high risk for breast cancer should consider not drinking alcohol at all).

Cervical Cancer

Cervical cancer is cancer that starts in the cervix, the lower part of the uterus (womb) that opens at the top of the vagina.

Cervical cancer usually develops very slowly. It starts as a precancerous condition called dysplasia. This precancerous condition can be detected by a Pap smear and is 100 percent treatable. It can take years for precancerous changes to turn into cervical cancer. Most women who are diagnosed with cervical cancer today have not had regular Pap smears or they have not followed up on abnormal Pap smear results.

Causes

Almost all cervical cancers are caused by HPV (human papilloma virus). HPV is a common virus that is spread through sexual intercourse. There are many different types of HPV. Some strains lead to cervical cancer. (Other strains may cause genital warts, while others do not cause any problems at all.)

A woman's sexual habits and patterns can increase her risk for cervical cancer. Risky sexual practices include having sex at an early age, having multiple sexual partners, and having multiple partners or partners who participate in high-risk sexual activities.

Common symptoms

Most of the time, early cervical cancer has no symptoms. Symptoms that may occur can include:

- Abnormal vaginal bleeding between periods, after intercourse, or after menopause.
- Continuous vaginal discharge, which may be pale, watery, pink, brown, bloody, or foul-smelling.
- Periods become heavier and last longer than usual.

Cervical cancer may spread to the bladder, intestines, lungs, and liver. Patients with cervical cancer do not usually have problems until the cancer is advanced and has spread. Symptoms of advanced cervical cancer may include:

- Back pain.
- Bone pain or fractures.
- Fatigue.
- Leaking of urine or faeces from the vagina.
- Leg pain.

- Loss of appetite.
- Pelvic pain.
- Single swollen leg.
- Weight loss.

Signs and tests

Precancerous changes of the cervix and cervical cancer cannot be seen with the naked eye. Special tests and tools are needed to spot such conditions.

- Pap smears screen for precancers and cancer, but do not make a final diagnosis.
- If abnormal changes are found, the cervix is usually examined under magnification. This is called colposcopy. Pieces of tissue are surgically removed (biopsied) during this procedure and sent to a laboratory for examination.
- Cone biopsy may also be done.

If the woman is diagnosed with cervical cancer, the health care provider will order more tests to determine how far the cancer has spread. This is called stageing. Tests may include:

- Chest x-ray.
- CT scan of the pelvis.
- Cystoscopy.
- Intravenous pyelogram (IVP).
- MRI of the pelvis.

Prevention

Practicing safe sex (using condoms) also reduces your risk of HPV and other sexually-transmitted diseases. HPV infection causes genital warts. These may be barely visible or several inches wide. If a woman sees warts on her partner's genitals, she should avoid intercourse with that person.

To further reduce the risk of cervical cancer, women should limit their number of sexual partners and avoid partners who participate in high-risk sexual activities.

Getting regular Pap smears can help detect precancerous changes, which can be treated before they turn into cervical cancer. Pap smears effectively spot such changes, but they must be done regularly. Annual pelvic examinations, including a pap smear, should start when a woman becomes sexually active, or by the age of 20 in a nonsexually active woman.

If you smoke, quit. Cigarette smoking is associated with an increased risk of cervical cancer.

Uterine Cancer

When Arushi Mittal, a stay-at-home wife, noticed that her bleeding wouldn't stop even after 20 days, she knew something wasn't right. An ultrasound confirmed her worst fears—she had uterine cancer! She had a long history of obesity and weighed 80 kilos for a 5'2" woman. Obesity is a strong risk factor for endometrial cancer (the most common type of uterine cancer and occurs in the inner lining of the uterus or the 'endometrium') because fatty tissues in women produce large amounts of estrogen. Overweight women are more likely than average to develop endometrial cancer. A diet high in fat can also be a risk factor.

Causes

Although the exact cause of endometrial cancer is unknown, increased levels of estrogen appear to play a role. Estrogen helps stimulate the buildup of the lining of the uterus. Studies have shown that high levels of estrogen in animals result in excessive endometrial growth and cancer.

Most cases of endometrial cancer occur between the ages of 60 and 70 years, but a few cases may occur before age 40.

Recent studies have seen that infertility boosts cancer risk, especially cancers of the uterus.

Causes and risk factors

The following increase your risk of endometrial cancer:

- Diabetes.
- Estrogen replacement therapy without the use of progesterone.
- History of endometrial polyps.
- Infertility (inability to become pregnant).
- Infrequent periods.
- Tamoxifen, a drug for breast cancer treatment.
- Never being pregnant.
- Obesity.
- Polycystic ovarian syndrome (PCOS).
- Starting menstruation at an early age (before age 12).
- Starting menopause after age 50.

Associated conditions include the following:

- Colon or breast cancer.
- Gallbladder disease.
- High blood pressure.

Common Symptoms

Symptoms of endometrial cancer include:

- Abnormal bleeding from the vagina, including bleeding between periods or spotting/bleeding after menopause.
- Extremely long, heavy, or frequent episodes of vaginal bleeding after age 40.
- Lower abdominal pain or pelvic cramping.
- Thin white or clear vaginal discharge after menopause.

Signs and tests

A pelvic examination is frequently normal, especially in the early stages of disease. Changes in the size, shape, or feel of the uterus or surrounding structures may be seen when the disease is more advanced.

Tests that may be done include:

- Endometrial aspiration or biopsy.
- Dilatation and curettage (D and C).
- Pap smear (may raise a suspicion for endometrial cancer, but does not diagnose it).

If cancer is found, other tests may be done to determine if the cancer has spread to other parts of the body. This is called stageing.

Complications

Complications may include anaemia due to blood loss. A perforation (hole) of the uterus may occur during a D and C or endometrial biopsy.

There can also be complications from hysterectomy, radiation, and chemotherapy.

Prevention

There is no effective screening test for endometrial (uterine) cancer. Women with any risk factors for endometrial cancer should be followed closely by their doctors. Frequent pelvic examinations and screening tests such as a Pap smear and endometrial biopsy may be considered in some cases.

Women who are taking estrogen replacement therapy without progesterone therapy or who have taken tamoxifen for more than 2 years have an increased risk of endometrial cancer and should have regular pelvic examinations and Pap smears.

Ovarian Cancer

Ovarian cancer is a cancerous growth arising from the ovary. Symptoms are frequently very subtle early on and may include: bloating, pelvic pain, difficulty eating and frequent urination, and are easily confused with other illnesses.

Time and again I have seen that this type of cancer goes unnoticed by women. They need to be aware if the signs and symptoms of such a type of cancer in order to catch it early. I remember this case of a particular patient of mine—Neeta. She would feel tired and stressed out most of the time. She was gaining weight at an alarming speed but would dismiss it as being inconsequential to pay notice. It was only when people around her started asking her if she was pregnant did she realize that her weight gain was, in fact, abnormal! A few routine tests confirmed she had stage-2 ovarian cancer.

Most (more than 90 percent) ovarian cancers are classified as 'epithelial' and are believed to arise from the surface of the ovary. However, some evidence suggests that the fallopian tube could also be the source of some ovarian cancers. Since the ovaries and tubes are closely related to each other, it is thought that these fallopian cancer cells can mimic ovarian cancer. Other types may arise from the egg cells (germ cell tumour) or supporting cells.

Causes

In most cases, the exact cause of ovarian cancer remains unknown. The risk of developing ovarian cancer appears to be affected by several factors.

- Older women who have never given birth, and those who have a first or second degree relative with the disease, have an increased risk.
- Hereditary forms of ovarian cancer can be caused by mutations in specific genes (most notably BRCA1 and BRCA2.
- Infertile women and those with a condition called endometriosis, and those who use postmenopausal estrogen replacement therapy are at increased risk.

A strong family history of uterine cancer, colon cancer, or other gastrointestinal cancers may indicate the presence of a syndrome known as hereditary nonpolyposis colourectal cancer (HNPCC, also known as Lunch Syndrome, which confers a higher risk for developing ovarian cancer).

Signs and symptoms

Signs and symptoms of ovarian cancer are frequently absent early on and when they exist they may be subtle. In most cases, the symptoms persist for several months before being recognized and diagnosed. Most typical symptoms include bloating, abdominal or pelvic pain, difficulty eating, and possibly urinary symptoms. If these symptoms recently started and occurs more frequently, the diagnosis should be considered.

Other findings include an abdominal mass, back pain, constipation, tiredness, and a range of other non-specific symptoms, as well as more specific symptoms such as abnormal vaginal bleeding or involuntary weight loss. There can be a build-up of fluid (ascites) in the abdominal cavity.

Ovarian cancer is associated with age, family history of ovarian cancer, anaemia, abdominal pain, abdominal distension, rectal bleeding, postmenopausal bleeding, loss of appetite, and weight loss.

Diagnosis

- Diagnosis of ovarian cancer starts with a physical examination (including a pelvic examination).
- A blood test (for CA-125 and sometimes other markers).
- Transvaginal ultrasound.
- The diagnosis must be confirmed with surgery to inspect the abdominal cavity, take biopsies (tissue samples formicroscopic analysis) and look for cancer cells in the abdominal fluid.

Conventional treatment

Treatment usually involves chemotherapy and surgery, and sometimes radiotherapy.

Complications

- Spread of the cancer to other organs.
- Progressive function loss of various organs.
- Ascites (fluid in the abdomen).
- Intestinal obstructions.

These cells can implant on other abdominal (peritoneal) structures, including the uterus, urinary bladder, bowel, lining of the bowel wall (omentum) and, less frequently, to the lungs.

Holistic approach to cancer

It aims to rejuvenate and detoxify the body. Specific immune boosters like wheatgrass juice, carrot juice, relaxation techniques like meditation, asana, pranayama, reflexology, acupressure, tranquilizing, and immune booster acupuncture points andwater therapies are beneficial. Ayurvedic treatments mainly help as a supportive which release the toxins and enhance the overall functioning of the organs.

Living a good healthy life, incorporating various aspects like diet, exercise, refraining from bad habits, regular health check-ups can all reduce the risk of breast cancer to a certain extent.

Treatment through holistic approach mainly is supportive. Allopathy is the choice to arrest the progress of the disease. But since the treatments like chemotherapy and radiation expose a person to various chemicals, toxicity sets in the body. Also the immunity is greatly suppressed. Holistic approach would be used to detoxify the system, thereby boosting the immunity. The healthy tissues and organs are rejuvenated and this helps fight against the spread of the disease to healthy tissues. We can de-stress the person, having gone through these difficult times, both physically and emotionally. Counselling is important to develop a positive attitude and to continue life, living healthily to the fullest.

Ayurvedic and homeopathic internal medications prevent the progression and to reverse the changes in the body.

Homeopathy

Homeopathy offers two modes of management for cancer cases. One is the constitutional approach where the cancer can go into remission and the metastasis (spread of cancer from one organ to the other) can be stopped from happening. Medicines like Natrum Muriaticum, Sepia, Ars Alb, and Thuja help. The other approach is supportive care where the metastasis has already happened. Here medicines like Kali Brom, Ars Alb, Conium, and Carbo Animalis help the patient.

Naturopathy

The aim is to detoxify the system and boost the immunity to arrest the progression of the disease. This is done through a disciplined diet, correcting bowel movements, and exercises to improve physical and mental health.

Ayurveda

Treatments are palliative, supportive, to de-stress, detoxify and to boost the immunity. Sirodhara is given to clear the emotions, calm the mind, and to rejuvenate. Choorna Swedam, Abhyanga, Navarakizhi, Pizhichil, and other special treatments are done to relieve the swelling and bodily discomfort, apart from improving the immunity and strength.

Treatments like Nasya, Vasti, Virechanam are done to de-toxify the system. Internal medications in the form of tablets, capsules and decoctions are prescribed to improve the immunity, strengthen the whole body and stop the progression and spread of the illness

Yoga

In general yogic postures help to keep one healthy. It does not play a special role in preventing cancer.

Diet

Ideally, a patient should exclude food containing phytoestrogesns like soya and its products, flaxseeds, elephant yam, fennel, and alfalfa.

COMMON MEDICAL CONDITIONS TREATABLE BY INTEGRATED MEDICINE

Circulatory System

- Anaemia
- Angina
- Aneurysm
- Athersclerosis
- Chilbains
- Enlarged spleen
- Gangrene
- Heart failure
- Hypertension (high blood pressure)
- Leukaemia
- Low blood pressure
- Palpitations
- Raynaud's disease
- Varicose veins

Respiratory System

- Asthma
- Catarrh
- Chronic bronchitis
- Common cold
- Coughs
- Emphysema
- Hay fever
- Hiccups
- Hyperventilation
- Influenza (Flu)
- Lung cancer
- Pleurisy
- Pneumonia
- Tracheitis
- Tuberculosis

Mind and Nervous System

- Anxiety
- Depression
- Depression
- Dizziness
- Encephalitis
- Epilepsy
- Fainting
- Headaches
- Insecurity
- Insomnia
- Memory Loss
- Meningitis
- Migraines
- Multiple sclerosis (MS)
- Neuralgia
- Obsessions and compulsions
- Parkinson's disease
- Phobias
- Repetitive strain injury (RSI)
- Shingles
- Stress
- Stroke

Digestive System

- Anal fissures
- Appendicitis
- Beer guts
- Cirrhosis of the liver
- Constipation
- Crohn's disease
- Diarrhoea
- Digestive cancers
- Flatulence and burping
- Gallstones
- Gastroenteritis
- Haemorrhoids
- Hepatitis
- Hernia
- Indigestion and heartburn

- ❖ Irritable bowel syndrome (IBS)
- ❖ Jaundice
- ❖ Liver problems
- ❖ Nausea and vomiting
- ❖ Obesity
- ❖ Pancreatitis
- ❖ Peptic ulcer
- ❖ Piles
- ❖ Travel sickness

Musculoskeletal System

- ❖ Arthritis
- ❖ Backache
- ❖ Breaks and fractures
- ❖ Bunions
- ❖ Bursitis
- ❖ Cramps
- ❖ Fibrositis
- ❖ Lumbago
- ❖ Muscular dystrophy
- ❖ Osteoporosis
- ❖ Rheumatism
- ❖ Sciatica
- ❖ Soft tissue damage
- ❖ Sprains and strains
- ❖ Tendinitis

Infants/Children

- ❖ Bedwetting
- ❖ Childhood leukaemia
- ❖ Chickenpox
- ❖ Chronic sleep disturbance
- ❖ Cold, Influenza
- ❖ Colic
- ❖ Constant crying
- ❖ Cough
- ❖ Cradle cap
- ❖ Croup
- ❖ Ear infections
- ❖ German measles (Rubella)
- ❖ Glue ear
- ❖ Hyperactivity
- ❖ Impetigo
- ❖ Measles
- ❖ Mumps
- ❖ Nappy rash
- ❖ Night terrors
- ❖ Sticky eye
- ❖ Teething
- ❖ Thrush (candidiasis)
- ❖ Vomiting and diarrhoea
- ❖ Whooping cough
- ❖ Worms

Endocrine System

- ❖ Addison's disease
- ❖ Diabetes
- ❖ Goitre
- ❖ Gout
- ❖ Hypoglycemia
- ❖ Obesity
- ❖ Thyroid problems

Immune (Lymphatic) System

- ❖ Allergies
- ❖ Glandular fever
- ❖ HIV and AIDS
- ❖ Hodgkin's disease
- ❖ ME (Myalgic Encephalomyelitis)

Male Reproductive System

- ❖ Cancer—Penile/Prostate/Testicular
- ❖ Ejaculation problems
- ❖ Erectile dysfunction
- ❖ Infertility
- ❖ Priapism
- ❖ Prostate problems
- ❖ Sexually transmitted diseases (STDs)

Female Reproductive System: Breast problems

- Breast-feeding problems
- Cancer—Cervical/Breast/Ovarian
- Childbirth
- Infertility
- Labour Pains
- Menopause
- Menstrual problems
- Miscarriage and abortions
- Ovarian cysts
- Painful intercourse
- Pelvic inflammatory diseases
- Post-delivery problems
- Postnatal depression
- Pregnancy
- Pre-menstrual syndrome
- Prolapse
- Sexually transmitted diseases (STDs)
- Thrush

Urinary System

- Cystitis (and bladder infection)
- Incontinence
- Kidney diseases
- Kidney stones
- Urethritis

Eyes

- Black eye
- Blepharitis
- Cataracts
- Conjunctivitis
- Eyestrain
- Glaucoma
- Squint
- Stye
- Twitching eyelids

Ears / Nose / Throat / Mouth

- Bad breath (Halitosis)
- Catarrh
- Cold Sores
- Dental Pain and phobia
- Ear ache
- Ear infection
- Ear wax
- Glue ear
- Gingivitis
- Laryngitis
- Mouth ulcers
- Nosebleeds
- Oral thrush
- Peridontal disease
- Sinus problems
- Sore throat
- Tinnitus
- Tonsillitis
- Toothache

Skin and Hair

- Abscesses
- Acne
- Athlete's foot
- Baldness
- Boils
- Cellulite
- Chilblains
- Cold sores
- Corns and calluses
- Dandruff
- Dermatitis
- Eczema
- Edema
- Excessive perspiration
- Hair loss
- Impetigo
- Prickly heat
- Psoriasis
- Ringworm
- Scabies
- Sunburn
- Urticaria
- Warts

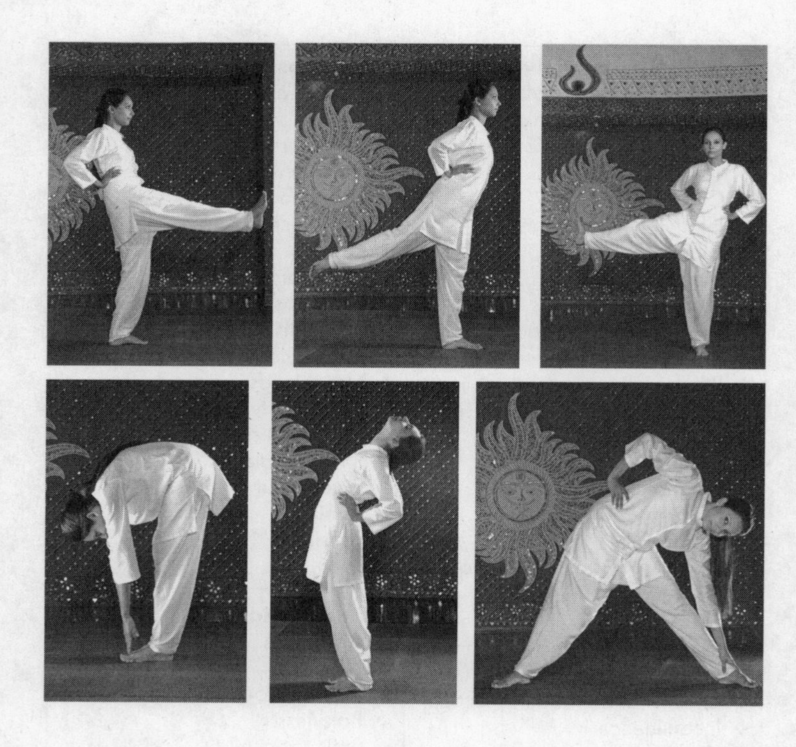

Hip Movements

- Slow and gentle rotation of the hips in both directions.
- Inhale and swing a leg forward, exhale and swing it backwards. Repeat from the other side, being aware of the stretch and compression felt in the hips.
- Inhale and lift the leg sideways up, and exhale and bring it down. Do it on the other side and feel the stretch.
- Backward bending from the hips as you inhale and forward bending as you exhale.
- Side tilts from both the sides as you exhale, inhale, and straighten.

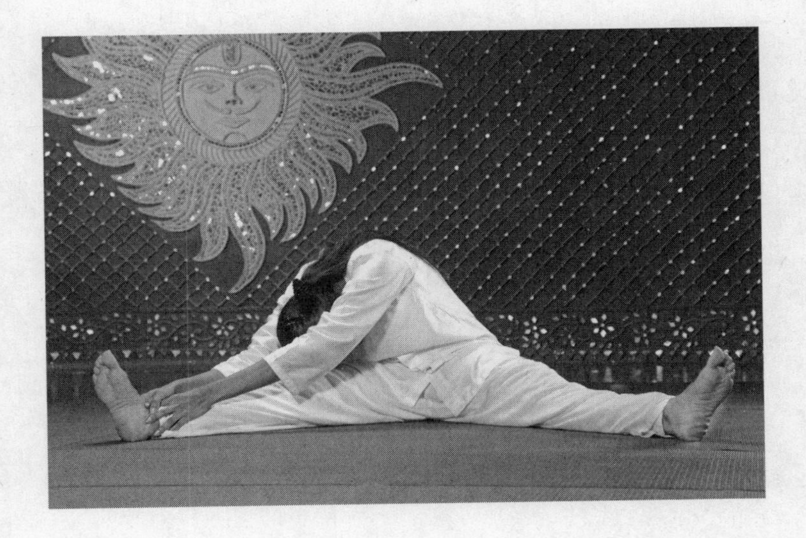

Janusirasana

- Bend your right knee and place it on the ground, such that the sole of the right foot touches the left inner thigh.
- Let the left leg be fully stretched.
- With an inhalation, raise your arms up.
- As you exhale, bend forward and hold the leg with your hands.
- You could either hold the ankles, the arch of your foot or the toes.
- As you continue normal breathing, with every exhalation, try and bend down further and if possible touch the forehead to the left knee.
- Feel the stretch in the hips and thighs.
- Feel the compression in the abdomen.
- Inhale; raise your arms up.
- Exhale; release them and extend the right leg.
- Relax for some time and repeat on the other side
- Relax in sitting position.

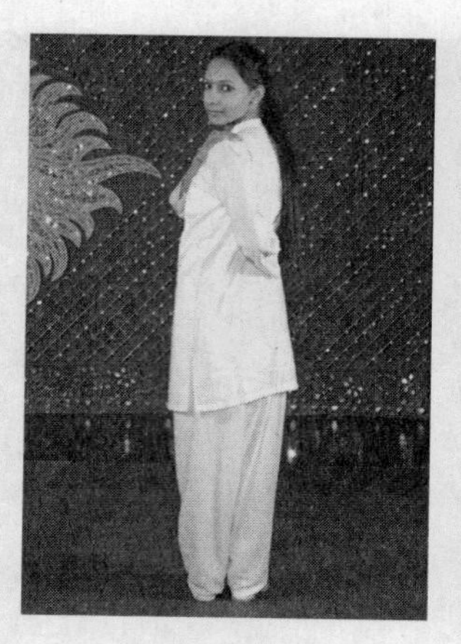
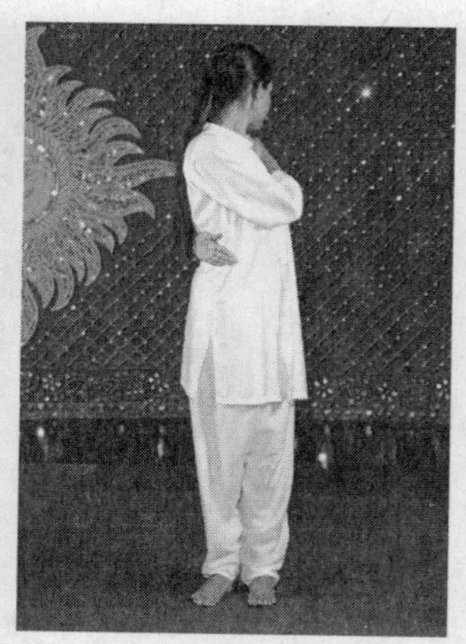

Kati Chakrasana

This is a spinal twisting posture.

- Stand with the feet together.
- Place the right hand on the left shoulder.
- Place the top of the left hand on the right hip, taking the arm across the spine.
- With an inhalation, twist the upper body to the left side and with the help of your right hand push the left shoulder.
- As you exhale, turn the head backwards.
- Breathe normally and hold the posture comfortably; be aware of the stretch you feel in the spine, shoulders, and hips.
- Enjoy the relaxation as you release the posture; Inhale turn the head forward, exhale and turn the upper body forwards.
- Repeat after complete relaxation on the other side of the body.

This asana could be done by people who have acute stiffness or pain in the back, without letting it aggravate.

Benefits

It relieves the stiffness from the spine, hips and shoulders • It relieves back pain • It has a stimulating effect on the digestive system, particularly the liver, kidneys, and spleen

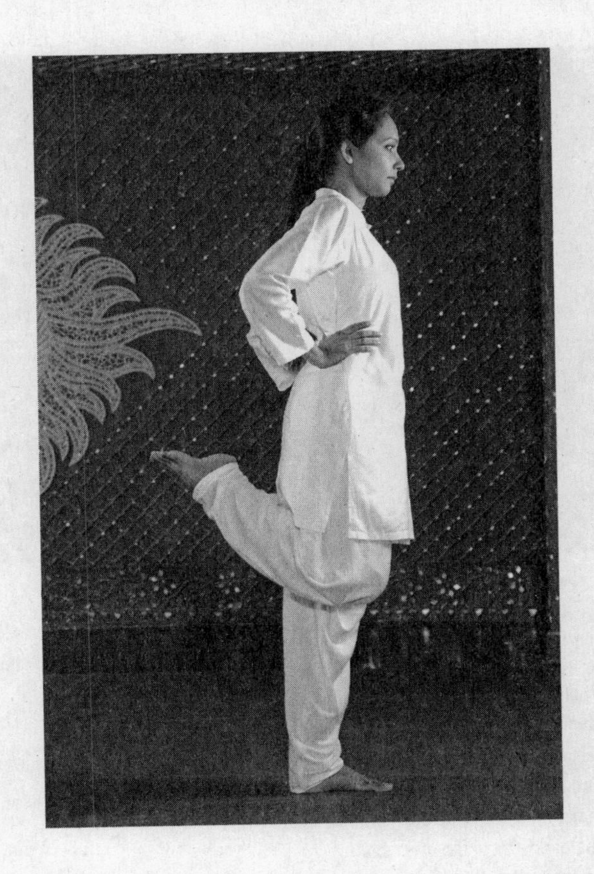

Knee Movements

Inhale and bend the knee backwards, exhale and stretch it. Repeat it on the other side

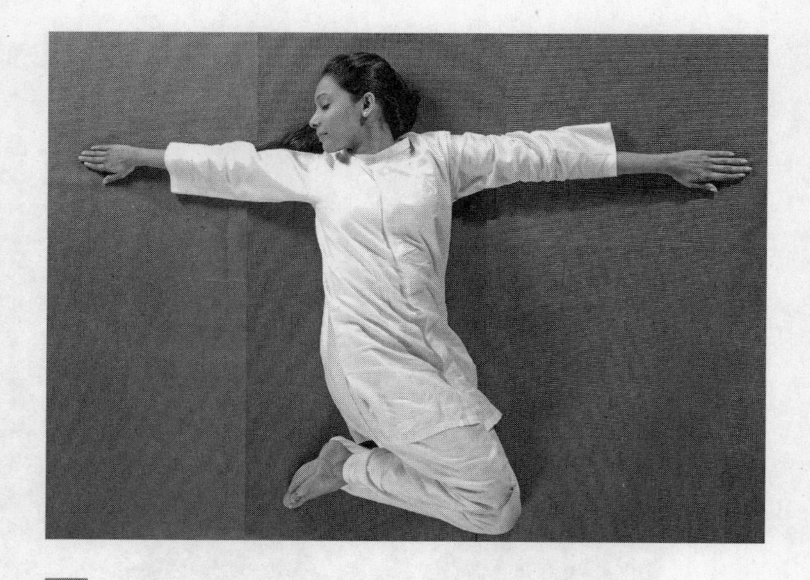

Makarabhyasa

- Lay on the back with the knees bent and feet placed on the ground.
- Extend the arms sideways at the shoulder level.
- Take a deep inhalation and as you exhale, tilt the knees to the left and turn the head to the right.
- Inhale; bring the head and knees back to centre.
- Exhale; now tilt to the other side.
- Repeat this few times.

Benefits

It stretches and relaxes the entire spine apart from improving the breath

Part II

Gynaecological Conditions

DO YOU KNOW WHEN TO SEE YOUR DOCTOR? CAN YOU recognize symptoms of a hormonal imbalance such as changes in menstruation, spotting, PMS, and delayed puberty? Do you ignore that constant ache in your back? Do you consult your pharmacist or your physician when you need to 'cure' a pain? Do you have severe menstrual cramps? Do you have a balanced diet? There are so many questions that, as a busy woman, you tend to leave unanswered, and would be relieved to forget about. This book will be the friend and guide you need to make sure you right the many wrongs your body has endured.

Frequently your doctor or you yourself may be tempted to resort to stop-gap measures such as the use of birth control pills to balance hormonal discrepancies. However, while the pill has its place in a woman's reproductive life, when used indiscriminately, for example to modify cycles to suit a modelling schedule, it can lead to future complications such as difficulties with conception and pregnancy.

The analogy of the birth control pill is used to illustrate the point that it is important to understand and be educated about the various medical options available to you and their potential side effects before accepting them as a form of treatment for a physiological condition.

CHAPTER FIVE

Menstrual Issues

DUE TO THE HORMONAL CHANGES A FEMALE BODY IS subjected to, there tend to be certain problems more frequently than others. They are flatulence, water retention, mood swings, stomach cramps, and anaemia apart from the symptoms during menopause like hot flashes, sleeplessness, and reduced calcium. Let's take a look at a few of them in detail.

Puberty

Puberty is the time when your body grows from a child's to an adult's. You'll know that you are going through puberty by the way your body changes.

If you're a girl, you'll notice that your breasts develop and your pubic hair grows, that you have a growth spurt, and that you get your period (menstruation). The overall shape of your body will probably change, too—your hips will widen and your body will become curvier.

If you're a boy, you'll start growing pubic and facial hair, have a growth spurt, and your testicles and penis will get larger. Your body shape will also begin to change—your shoulders will widen and your body will become more muscular.

These changes are caused by the sex hormones (testosterone in boys and estrogen in girls) that your body begins producing in much larger amounts than before.

Puberty takes place over a number of years, and the age at which it starts and ends varies widely. It generally begins somewhere between the ages of 7 and 13 for girls, and somewhere between the ages of 9 and 15 for boys, although it can be earlier or later for some people. This wide range in age is normal, and it's why you may develop several years earlier (or later) than most of your friends.

Causes

Causes of delayed or abnormal puberty can be any of the following:

- Constitutional delay in growth and puberty (CDGP)—sporadic or familial.
- Chronic illness, eg. kidney disease, Crohn's disease.
- Malnutrition, eg. anorexia nervosa, cystic fibrosis, coeliac disease.
- Excessive physical exercise, particularly athletes or gymnasts.
- Psychosocial deprivation.
- Steroid therapy.
- Hypothyroidism.
- Trauma: surgery, head injury.
- Various hormonal and genetic disorders.

Examination

Examine the height, weight, and any signs that look suspicious of malnutrition. Try to compare the height and weight of parents and siblings with the individual's.

Investigations

They could be conducted through appropriate blood tests to assess the level of hormones. If needed, scans are done to assess the condition of internal organs and malfunctions if any.

Management

First and foremost, it is important to build the confidence in the child and give her all the moral support. This is the period in which the child would be embarrassed and ashamed to interact socially. He could be teased by his friends at school too. Counselling by elders is needed at this point.

Elaborate tests should be done as per the guidance of physicians to rule out involvement of major hormones. Medications should be started to improve the secretions if needed. Diet should be focussed on too. Nutritious food can help the organs function better and help the growth.

Holistic approach

Homeopathy

A constitutional approach has to be taken in conditions of delayed puberty in young girls. The treatment will be addressing the root cause of the complaint.

Naturopathy

Treatments to stimulate the production of hormones could be done which would include hydrotherapy, massage, and acupuncture apart from the diet.

Ayurveda

It has very good medications to stimulate the body's natural rhythm. If needed, treatments like Sirodhara, and Abhyanga help too.

Yoga

Exercises including yogic techniques like pranayama and meditation helps too.

Bodily Changes with Puberty

The bodily changes with puberty happen when a child grows and becomes an adult. The body secretes hormones which bring on these changes, often very quickly. This is when the body matures and reaches puberty. It is a transitional phase.

Girls grow taller, their shoulders and hips may broaden, and they could put on weight for a while. There will be changes in the breast, development of hairs in the underarms, pubic region, around vulva, and also more hair on arms and legs or around nipples. The voice gets a bit deeper, though not as noticeably as a boy's does. Hair and skin might get oily and one might get pimples though those won't last forever. There will be the onset of the menstrual cycles. The regular menstrual cycle is once every 28–30 days. One would bleed for 5–6 days. Spotting could continue for a day or two more.

Girls also notice a white, odourless vaginal discharge in-between the periods. This is a normal, physiological secretion. But if this gets profuse, with curd-like or thick consistency, with a yellowish tinge or with strong foul smell, it's a sign of infection and should be treated accordingly. This could also lead to itching at times.

Holistic approach

Homeopathy

Bodily changes in puberty can cause confusion and worry in children. Medicines like Natrum Mur, Ignatia, Pulsatilla, and Staphysagria can help the adolescents.

Yoga

Yoga is a complete form of exercise and hence incorporating various forms of yoga like the asanas, pranayamas, and meditation along with the relaxation techniques help in overall personality development.

One should try and start off the day with exercise, at least for 45 minutes. If it's absolutely not possible in the mornings, then one could choose an ideal time of the day, except immediately after a meal. A gap of at least 2 hours should be given between a meal and exercise.

Diet

Puberty is the time when the body starts showing changes and develops into adulthood. This is the time when the reproductive system, the endocrines, the musculoskeletal system, and the body as a whole undergo changes. One has a high metabolic rate. Digestion is at its peak. One's appearance undergoes a change. Mentally, there is a lot of conflict, as one neither considers themselves a child, nor do they have the maturity of an adult.

This is the time of maximum growth. The diet should be wholesome with adequate quantities of all the vital nutrients.

- Protein intake is the most important. Proteins should be supplemented through good sources like chicken without skin, fish, egg whites, lentils and pulses, milk and its products, and soya milk.
- Carbohydrates should be included through rice, wheat, oats, ragi, bajra, and jowar. These should be taken for breakfast, lunch, and dinner. It is healthier to take them in steamed form, roasted snacks, as porridge, or as bread made with a combination of these grains/flour.
- Underground vegetables like potato, sweet potato, yam, and colocasia are also good sources of carbohydrates and fibre.
- Fat consumption should also be high during this period. Healthy sources of fat are whole milk, vegetable oils, pure cow's ghee, cod liver oil, oil from fish, and nuts.

- Vitamins and minerals can be supplied through green leafy vegetables, coloured vegetables, fruits, dry fruits, and nuts.
- Trace elements like zinc, selenium, copper, iron are also very important apart from calcium, potassium, and sodium. These could be supplemented through wholesome and healthy eating.
- Iron deficiency (anaemia) is common during this period because of the blood loss during menstruation. One should supplement iron through dates, black raisins, leafy vegetables, beetroot, and palm jaggery.
- Calcium should be supplemented through milk and its products, ragi, soya, spinach, chicken, and fish.
- Water intake should be adequate. One should drink upto 3 litres of water as all the metabolic activities need water as a medium. One can also drink unsweetened fruit and vegetable juices, butter milk, lime water, coconut water and herbal teas to keep the system hydrated.
- One can go in for healthier versions like wholewheat bread, wholewheat pizza, noodles and pasta, multigrain biscuits, and oats biscuits. Also the fillings and toppings could be made healthier by avoiding mayonnaise and cheese and going in for cottage cheese instead, opting for grilled/ baked patties instead of the deep fried ones.
- Breakfast is the first meal of the day, after long hours of starvation. This meal should never be skipped. Breakfast should be wholesome containing cereals or bread, fruits or juices, egg, etc. It should provide the energy needed to start the day's activities.
- If there is an opportunity for a mid-morning snack, it is ideal. One could take some nuts or dry fruits or fresh fruits or roasted grams.
- Lunch can be moderate with bread or rice accompanied by vegetables, lentils, curd or buttermilk, chicken or fish.
- One should take a mid-afternoon snack, which could again

be some salads, fruits, sprouts, smoothies, and crackers.

- Dinner should be light with smaller quanties of food. Make sure you do not completely fill the stomach at dinner.
- If one is in the habit of studying late into night, then it would be good to have some fruits 3–4 hours after dinner, to give the energy to continue studying.
- Skipping meals is a common trend seen in adolescents. This should never be encouraged. It would be reflected in the general state of health and the level of energy, intelligence, concentration, and memory.
- One reason for doing it is to stay slim. But the fact is that the nutritional status is highly compromised, reflecting on the skin, reproductive system, digestive system and the mental and emotional health.
- Junk food includes deep fried food, food made of white flour and refined products, food with additives and preservatives, aerated drinks, food with lot of cheese, butter, and mayonnaise. These should be avoided.
- Eating junk and skipping meals could be the cause of acne, dry skin, hair loss, acidity, gastritis, constipation, menstrual irregularities, and sometimes infertility.
- It could also turn into psychosomatic issues like bulimia and anorexia nervosa.

DR MATHAI'S TIPS

- Along with proper diet, exercise too plays a great role. Since most youngsters prefer staying indoors, mostly with computers and indoor games, physical activity is minimal. A conscious effort should be made to exercise regularly. Any form of exercise is ideal. Walking, jogging, swimming, dance forms, gym, and yoga are all good.

- Regular exercising improves blood circulation, tones the muscles, improves the flexibility of joints, strengthens bones, and stimulates the internal organs. It also helps improve posture. It builds confidence in a person, improves memory, and concentration. The skin breathes better and stays beautiful.
- Regular exercise also helps the release of serotonin, a neuro- chemical which stabilizes the mood. It helps a person stay calm.

Hair Growth on the Body

The normal amount of body hair for women varies. Most of the time, a woman only has fine hair, above the lips and on the chin, chest, abdomen, or back. If one has coarse, dark hairs in these areas, the condition is called hirsutism. Such hair growth is more typical of men.

Causes

Women normally produce low levels of male hormones (androgens). If a body produces too much of this hormone, one may have unwanted hair growth.

In most cases, the exact cause is never identified. It tends to run in families. In general, hirsutism is a harmless condition. But many women find it bothersome, or even embarrassing.

A common cause of hirsutism is polycystic ovarian syndrome (PCOS). Women with PCOS and other hormone conditions that cause unwanted hair growth may also have acne, problems with menstrual periods, trouble losing weight, and diabetes. Other, rare causes of unwanted hair growth may include:

- Tumour or cancer of the adrenal gland.
- Tumour or cancer of the ovary.
- Cushing syndrome.
- Congenital adrenal hyperplasia.
- Hyperthecosis (a condition in which the ovaries produce too much male hormones).
- Use of certain medicines, including testosterone.

Prevention

Hirsutism is generally a long-term problem. There are a number of ways to remove or treat unwanted hair. Some treatment effects last longer than others.

- Weight loss in overweight women can reduce hair growth.
- Bleaching or lightening hair may make it less noticeable.

Temporary hair removal options include:

- Shaving does not cause more hair to grow, but the hair may look thicker.
- Plucking and waxing are fairly safe and not expensive. However, they can be painful and there is a risk for scarring, swelling, and skin darkening. Sometimes chemicals are used in these procedures which could cause some skin damage.

One should seek a medical professional if the hair grows rapidly, or if the girl has other features such as acne, deepening voice, increased muscle mass, and decreased breast size.

Holistic approach

The holistic approach for hirsuitism mainly aims to treat the root cause for such development. Through detailed evaluation, examination, and necessary lab investigations, we elicit the root cause and treat it accordingly.

Internal medications are given to regularize the hormones. External treatments from ayurveda and naturopathy leads to internal cleansing which leads to proper functioning of all the organs and systems, including the hormone secretions.

Shirodhara helps in hormone regulation. Choorna Swedam helps open up the channels and detoxify the system.

Homeopathy

Graphites, Sepia, Lycopodium, Thuja are some of the homeopathic medicines used for excessive hair growth on body. These medicines should be taken in consultation with a homeopathic physician.

Naturopathy

- Some of the natural products used to remove hair are a paste of chickpea flour and turmeric powder. This should be applied on the hairy part and left until it dries fully. Later you can just rub off the dried paste with your bare hands and fine hair is removed.
- A mixture of lemon juice and honey applied regularly can give a bleaching effect and lighten the hair.

Ayurveda

Ayurvedic treatments like Sirodhara, Abhyanga etc. help to regularize the hormones and thereby control the excessive hair growth.

Painful Menstruation

Painful menstrual periods cause a woman to have crampy lower abdominal pain, sharp or aching pain that comes and goes, or possibly back pain. Although some pain during the period is normal, excessive pain is not. The medical term for painful menstrual periods is dysmenorrhoea. As many as half of menstruating women are affected by dysmenorrhoea, and of these, about 10 percent have severe dysmenorrhoea, which greatly limits activities for 1–3 days each month.

It can feature different kinds of pain, including sharp, throbbing, dull, nauseating, burning, or shooting pain. Dysmenorrhoea may precede menstruation by several days or may accompany it, and it usually subsides as menstruation tapers off.

The main symptom is pain concentrated in the lower abdomen, in the umbilical region. It is also commonly felt in the right or left abdomen. It may radiate to the thighs and lower back. Symptoms often begin immediately following ovulation and can last until the end of menstruation. This is because it is often associated with changes in hormonal levels in the body that occur with ovulation.

Symptoms of vomiting, diarrhoea, and headache sometimes accompany menstruation, which are also included in dysmenorrhoea.

Prevention

- Apply a heating pad to your lower abdomen area, below your belly button.
- Light circular massage with your fingertips around your lower abdomen area can help.
- Drink warm beverages.
- Eat light but frequent meals.
- Follow a diet rich in carbohydrates such as whole grains, fruits, and vegetables, but low in salt, sugar, alcohol, and caffeine.
- Keep your legs raised while lying down, or lie on your side with your knees bent.
- Practice relaxation techniques such as meditation or yoga.
- Take warm showers or baths.
- Walk or exercise regularly, including pelvic rocking exercises.

- Lose weight if you are overweight.
- Omega-3 fatty acids that are found in fish such as salmon, mackerel, sardines, and anchovies help in this situation. They are also available in fish oil capsules, which may be the preferable form. Nuts and seeds too have omega-3 fatty acids.
- Magnesium is a mineral found naturally in foods such as green leafy vegetables, nuts, seeds, and whole grains. Magnesium is needed for more than 300 biochemical reactions in the body.

Holistic approach

A holistic approach should be taken with attention to diet and lifestyle as well as medication. Regular exercise helps to reduce the severity of symptoms while both smoking and passive inhalation of cigarette smoke increase the severity of these symptoms. Treatments are aimed to reduce discomfort and pain. It includes Sirodhara, Abhyanga, herbal hip bath, enema, mud packs, acupuncture, and acupressure.. Regular practice of yoga with pranayama and relaxation techniques also helps in this condition.

Hydrotherapy like compresses, hip baths, arm and foot bath help reduce the uterine spasms and hence the pain.

Reflexology, acupressure, and a hot foot immersion helps to relax and manage pain better.

Application of castor oil on the abdomen followed by hot fomentation also helps.

A relaxing massage with oil containing mint or camphor can ease the pain.

Internal medications from ayurveda and homeopathy help too.

A decoction made with roasted cumin seeds in water, helps to reduce the flatulence and induce uterine contractions. This ensures painless menstruation.

Homeopathy

Colocynth 30 taken frequently will help in easing the cramps during menstruation. Magnesium phosphoricum 3x 8 pills should be mixed in warm water and sipped frequently as they will help in reducing the pain. Caulophyllum 30 is also a good remedy for pain during menstruation when there is severe pain in the back also.

Ayurveda

Medicines like Saptasaram Kashayam, Lodhrasavam, Sukumaram Kashayam, and Kumariasavam help along with treatments like Yoni Pichu, Vasti, and Abhyanga.

Irregular Menstruation

Before we can define an irregular period, we must first determine what a regular period is. People often say that a regular period occurs every 28 days, but actually, every woman's menstrual cycle is different. Depending on the body and hormones, one may get a period every 20 days or you may get your period every 35 days. A good way to determine if your periods are regular is to keep a chart and count the number of days between each period. If they occur with roughly the same number of days between each cycle, then your periods are regular. A regular period typically lasts 5 days, but it is completely normal to menstruate for anywhere between 3 and 7 days.

Irregular periods aren't unusual. They affect about 30 percent of women in their reproductive years. An irregular period is any type of bleeding that is abnormal when compared to a usual menstrual cycle. This can include a late period, an early period, or bleeding between periods. It can also appear as particularly heavy bleeding or scanty bleeding. Many women also experience irregular periods in the form of a missed period, continuous periods, or periods that occur twice in one cycle.

Causes

Irregular menstrual periods are usually the result of hormonal signals that have been thrown out of sync. In order to produce a period, the body makes hormones like estrogen and progesterone. These hormones are kept in the hypothalamus, pituitary gland, and ovaries inside your body. In order to trigger ovulation and menstruation, these parts of the body need to send signals to one another. Sometimes, these signals get crossed or skipped, causing irregular periods.

There are actually a number of things that can easily cause hormone levels to change.

- ❖ Pregnancy: If you are pregnant, your body will begin producing different levels of hormones. This will cause numerous pregnancy symptoms, including an end to your period.
- ❖ Stress: Stress is a common cause of irregular periods. If you are fatigued, worried, or anxious, it can cause your hormones to become unbalanced.
- ❖ Diet: A poor diet or extreme weight loss or gain can also affect your hormones. Women with anorexia or bulimia often have no period or irregular periods. Simple anaemia too causes irregular periods.
- ❖ Exercise: Intense exercise can wreak havoc on your body, often causing irregular periods.
- ❖ Menarche: The cycles after a girl's first period may be irregular for some time. It can take up to 3 years to get regular periods.
- ❖ Menopause: Menopause causes changes in your hormone levels, and is often signalled by irregular periods.
- ❖ Hormonal birth control: Birth control pills and irregular

periods sometimes go hand in hand. It can take a while for your body to adjust to the new levels of hormones delivered by hormonal birth control.

For most women, an irregular period is nothing to be worried about; a majority of women will eventually develop a regular cycle with regular periods. Sometimes though, underlying complications can be the cause of these period problems. If you are noticing particularly irregular periods, or have gone a year or more with missed periods, see your doctor. If you experience extreme cramping, heavy period bleeding, dizziness, nausea, or fainting, you should visit your healthcare provider.

Prevention

Treatments are done depending on the cause of irregular periods. If you have only been experiencing irregular periods for a short time (less than 7 months), it is likely that your periods will become regular again on their own. However, if there is an underlying medical condition that is causing your irregular periods, then receiving treatment for the condition should help to get periods back on track.

- Reduce your stress levels. Take time to meditate and relax. This may help put your cycle back on track.
- Get help for your eating disorder. If you are anorexic, bulimic, or if you suffer from other types of disordered eating, you must seek help. Not only will these eating disorders interrupt your menstrual cycle, they can also severely affect your liver, bowel, throat, and heart functions.
- Don't over-exercise. While it is important to exercise regularly and keep fit, exercising too much can be problematic. If you are an endurance athlete, try to cut back on your training a little bit, until your irregular periods return to normal.

Holistic approach

Holistic approach plays a very beneficial role in treating such conditions.

Homeopathy

The cause for irregular menstruation should be ascertained. The patient has to go through a thorough homeopathic evaluation by a homeopathic physician. However constitutional medicines like Pulsatilla, Sepia, Lachysis, Graphitis, and Calcarea Carb are helpful.

Naturopathy

Naturopathic therapies like hip bath, wet packs, yoga, meditation techniques, acupuncture for hormonal imbalance, and a specific diet are the major line of treatments. Internal herbal and homeopathic medicines are also needed.

Ayurveda

Ayurvedic therapies like Panchakarma, Sirodhara, Choorna Swedam, Abhyanga, herbal hip bath, Nasyam can help to regulate the imbalances in hormone levels and thus regulating the periods.

Yoga

Yoga is a proven effective method in regularizing the hormones and helping regular menstruation.

Diet

Eating papaya, til seeds, and palm jaggery helps to get periods, if they are delayed.

Hygiene

It is important to maintain proper hygiene especially after puberty, as there are body secretions which give rise to infections, if not cleaned properly. Sexual hygiene is also equally important.

Bodily secretions like the sweat, vaginal discharge etc. can give rise to fungal infections if not cleaned properly. Other than affecting externally, it could also get internal and affect the organs, sometimes leading to permanent damage.

Sometimes painful cysts develop, needing an incision. These could also get recurrent in nature.

There are also instances where these infections have lead to tubal block causing infertility.

One could experience severe itching, foul smelling discharge, and burning sensation with urination.

Prevention

- Starts with the oral hygiene. The trouble with the teeth and gums usually start with puberty. There could be bad breath, painful tooth and gums, caries and cavities etc. One should surely brush their teeth twice a day. Any infection should immediately be attended to.
- The fungus could attack the nails, skin, and scalp. Care should be taken to keep them clean and dry. Natural scrubs and cleansers with green gram, turmeric etc. could be used to keep the skin healthy. The scalp should be cleaned with soap nut or extract of hibiscus leaves. Applying lemon juice mixed with warm coconut oil on the scalp prevents dandruff. Nails should be protected well too with regular trimming and by cleaning the dirt that collects at the corners. They should be cleaned properly with soap and water.

- The hair from the axilla (underarms) and the pubic region should be removed or trimmed regularly. Excessive hair could create an ideal condition for the growth of organisms. One should do it with care, with antiseptic precautions.
- The private parts should be cleaned thoroughly after urinating and defecating. Too much usage of soap could lead to dryness and itchiness. Cleaning with lukewarm plain water is the best. After defecating, one should never wipe forwards, as it could contaminate the pubic region and cause infection.
- Bathing twice a day, changing the undergarments twice a day, and washing it thoroughly and sun drying it before next use are all a part of the routine hygiene measures and can reduce the chance of infections.

Holistic approach

Homeopathy

The homeopathic medicine Sulphur is good for people who do not maintain hygiene or for people who hate to take baths. Psorinum is a good remedy which can be given for lack of hygiene or for having bad body odour.

Naturopathy

- Naturopathy advices the use of neem decoctions to wash the private parts.
- Rinse the mouth with a decoction of mint leaves and few leaves of neem to arrest infection and give fresh breath.
- Brushing with neem twigs at least once a day also helps.

Ayurveda

- Washing the private parts with a decoction of triphala is recommended.
- Gargling the mouth with yastimadhu and turmeric

decoction helps.

- Bathing with water which has drops of lemon juice and vertiver added will give freshness and remove body odour.

White Discharge

The vagina serves as a passageway between the outside of the body and the inner reproductive organs. The pH balance of the vagina is acidic, which discourages infections from occurring. This acidic environment is created by normally-occurring bacteria. A healthy vagina produces secretions to cleanse and regulate itself, similar to how saliva cleanses and regulates the environment of the mouth. These vaginal secretions are normal vaginal discharge. Any interference with the delicate balance of vaginal secretions sets up an environment conducive to infection.

Normal vaginal discharge

All women have some vaginal discharge. Normal discharge may appear clear, cloudy white, and/or yellowish when dry on clothing. It may also contain white flecks and at times may be thin and stringy. Changes in normal discharge can occur for many reasons, including menstrual cycle, emotional stressors, nutritional status, pregnancy, usage of medications (including birth control pills), and sexual arousal.

Effects of the menstrual cycle

The menstrual cycle affects the vaginal environment. One may notice increased wetness and clear discharge around mid-cycle. The pH balance of the vagina fluctuates during the cycle and is the least acidic on the days just prior to and during menstruation. Infections, therefore, are most common at this time.

Common causes of abnormal discharge

There are many possible causes of abnormal vaginal discharge, but it is usually a sign of infection. The infection is often caused by something that upsets the natural balance of bacteria or yeast in the vagina, such as washing inside the vagina, or it may be sexually transmitted.

The most common causes are:

- Thrush—a fungal infection that commonly affects the vagina.
- Bacterial vaginosis—a bacterial infection of the vagina.
- Trichomoniasis—a sexually transmitted infection (STI) caused by a tiny parasite.
- Gonorrhoea or chlamydia—STIs caused by bacteria.
- Genital herpes—an STI caused by the herpes simplex virus.

Types

It is unusual for young girls to have abnormal vaginal discharge before they have gone through puberty. Abnormal discharge is also unusual in older women. If you have gone through the menopause and suddenly notice an abnormal vaginal discharge, see your doctor as soon as possible to rule out cervical cancer or endometrial cancer.

Watery or white vaginal discharge with intense itchiness

If the discharge is thin and watery or thick and white (like cottage cheese), the patient may have thrush. This common fungal infection causes intense itchiness and soreness around vagina. The discharge may smell slightly yeasty, but does not have a strong smell.

Almost all women get thrush from time to time and it is not sexually transmitted.

White or grey fishy-smelling discharge

If the vaginal discharge is grey or develops a strong fishy smell, particularly after sexual intercourse, one could have bacterial vaginosis (BV). BV is an imbalance in the normal bacteria found in the vagina. It does not usually cause itching or irritation.

Like thrush, BV is very common and is not sexually transmitted.

Green, yellow, or frothy discharge

Trichomoniasis is a common STI caused by a tiny parasite. It can make the vaginal discharge frothy, yellow, or green. One may have a lot of discharge, which may also have an unpleasant fishy smell. Other possible symptoms are soreness, swelling and itching around the vagina, and pain when passing urine.

Abnormal discharge with pain or bleeding

If the vaginal discharge is abnormal and associated with pain in pelvis or during urination, or you bleed between periods or after sex, one may have chlamydia or gonorrhoea (both STIs). Gonorrhoea can make the discharge turn green, although often the pain or bleeding is more noticeable. Untreated gonorrhoea or chlamydia may spread upwards and lead to pelvic inflammatory disease, a serious infection of the womb, fallopian tubes, or ovaries.

Abnormal discharge with blisters around the genitals

Genital herpes can cause painful, red blisters or sores to appear around your genitals, as well as an abnormal vaginal discharge.

Holistic approach

Homeopathic and ayurvedic internal medicines are most

beneficial. These medications mainly aim at maintaining the ph of the mucosa, so as to help prevent infections. The growth of the organism, if any, is arrested.

Homeopathy

Kreosote can help in white discharge with itching in vagina. Pulsatilla, Sepia, Natrum Mur, and Acid Nit are some of the constitutional homeopathic medicines to treat white discharge or leucorrhoea.

Naturopathy

Naturopathic therapies like vaginal douche, wet packs, and herbal hip baths are most beneficial in treating vaginal discharge.

Ayurveda

Ayurvedic treatments like vaginal douche with triphala decoction helps relive infection, maintain the pH of the mucosa, and reduce itchiness.

Spices like mustard, chilli, black pepper should be avoided. Cooling foods like tender coconut water, banana, sarsaparilla, and arrow root are advised.

Medications like Muesli Kadiradi Kashayam, Satavarigulam, and Chandanasavam are advised.

Lifestyle management through proper hygiene, healthy food intake etc. to prevent and deal with infections is also beneficial.

Behaviour with Opposite Sex and Peer Pressure

During adolescence, one becomes conscious about oneself. The innocence of childhood is lost partially, and one becomes aware of his appearance, the need to be recognized, the need to be on par with peers, and also certain normal human feelings such as jealousy, greed etc. sets in. There are a lot of bodily changes too at this time. One starts looking at the opposite sex with a different view. Feelings of infatuation and love set in. One starts getting interested in knowing more about sex. Feelings of anger, irritability, and restlessness and the '1 know all' attitude is prominent during adolescence.

With all these changes, even peer pressure is high. Comparisons start at various levels.

There are comparisons in studies, at home, in looks, and in relationships.

Few aspects generally compared to or mocked at are the height, weight, skin texture, hair (even bodily hair), mental sharpness, style of walking, and style of speaking.

Being constantly compared, and not being able to perform up to expectations, not having good friends, not being attractive —especially to the opposite sex—can cause a lot of emotional disturbances. This could affect the confidence, concentration, and self-esteem of the child. There are also instances where these have lead to depression and social withdrawal.

This is also the time when one would want to experiment and experience various things in life. What actually starts as fun or experimentation could lead to some dangerous results, especially, experimenting with alcohol, drugs, and smoking. If one has a tendency towards addiction, this experimentation would be enough to make them an addict as well.

First and foremost one needs to understand that no two individuals are the same. Each person is different in totality, even two siblings.

The way one looks, feels, responds, studies, and behaves are all her personal qualities and one can never be compared. But on a few aspects, changes could be made voluntarily after some self-realization or after being told by other people.

One needs to be confident about oneself. Look at all the good qualities in you and appreciate them. This can boost your feeling of self-worth.

Likewise, look at the negatives in you and try to make changes wherever possible, without being too harsh on yourself. There are certain things you cannot change, however hard you try. This could simply be because you were born with that trait. Try to accept those things. Believing in your own worth and not letting other's behaviour or attitude affect you is important.

Generally groups tend to form very quickly in schools. Groups are formed either by like-minded people or through chance meetings. One should be intuitive enough to choose the right group of friends. If someone accidentally falls into the wrong company, they should have the willingness and courage to break through.

Friends have to be chosen based on their honesty, good habits, behaviour, sincerity, and faithfulness. Friends should be with you at good and bad times alike. The same way, your approach to them should also make them consider and care for you.

In true friendships, gender does not matter. Most often, we see better friendships among people of the opposite sex.

Unfortunately during this period, one tends to consider their friends to be above their parents. They think parents are from an earlier generation and they know very little about today's world. They think that friends know better. The fact that parents and elders have seen the world for longer and have experienced more tricky situations, and their judgments can be valued better, is forgotten or ignored. Children tend to forget that their friends belong to the same age as them and their knowledge and abilities are limited, and hence relying on their opinions and judgments might not be the best idea.

Falling in so called 'love' also happens in adolescence. Most of these relationships are short-lived. It is considered healthy when one starts to get those feelings towards people of the opposite sex. It shows that the hormones are secreting in the right way. One should also know the difference between the right touch and the wrong one. Merely through a glance or touch one can understand the motive behind it. This cannot be taught practically, but being aware and cautious can definitely help.

This wrong touch could be even from the most unexpected relationships like teachers, uncles, siblings, or even fathers. (Yes, it's unbelievable, but true. And such incidents are getting more and more frequent, unfortunately.)

Often friendships turn into love affairs. There are cases where the friends tease two individuals and as a result they end up 'being in love'. Sometimes its mere infatuation leading to relationship. At times it's also to prove to peers that one is attractive or capable of being in a relationship. At this point they are too young to recognize the right qualities in an individual. It is superficial and ends up being physical too easily as well. This physical attraction can also be misused by the partner in various ways these days. Some lives are ruined completely because of such situations.

So in difficult situations, or when you are in trouble, rather than discussing it among your friends, it's best to share it with your parents or trusted elders. If you happen to commit a mistake, knowingly or unknowingly, parents—especially your mother—are the best people you can share these things with. They will always show you the right path and will only do the best for you without letting you get hurt in any way. In fact they are the only ones who care about you the most and mean the best.

As an individual too, one should be strong enough to react in the best way possible when injustice is done to you, whatever way it may be.

At school, teachers play the role of caretakers. One should not be apprehensive to expose those who trouble or bully you. It's a general fear, that one would be left alone, if they complaine about someone. That is temporary and by not bring it to the attention of elders, one is helping those bullies grow.

Medical attention could be sought, in reversing medically treatable conditions. Counselling, if needed, could be done to overcome the fears, troubles, and inhibitions of adolescence. This could be through professionals or through experienced elders.

Holistic approach

Homeopathy

Pulsatilla is a good medicine for fear of men in females. There are also other constitutional medicines like Sepia, Staphysagria etc. These medicines are to be given on the basis of symptom totality and not on the basis of fear alone. Hence consultation with a homeopathic physician is a must if there is any behavioural problem with the opposite sex.

Yoga

Yoga is the best tool for personality development. Yoga asanas and suryanamaskars help mould one's physical self. Body sculpting can be done through yogic postures. Pranayama, meditation, and deep relaxation techniques help one get better mentally and emotionally. Concentration, focus, intelligence, and memory get better with the regular practice of these techniques.

Special techniques like Trataka (candle meditation), and yoga nidra are the best tools to improve concentration and relax and sharpen the mind.

Urinary Incontinence

Urinary incontinence is defined as the involuntary urination because of loss of bladder control. It is a common and embarrassing problem which affects the quality of life.

Causes

The common causes are age, relaxed pelvic floor muscles, chronic cough, as a symptom of UTI, multiple pregnancies, diabetes mellitus, and prostate enlargement in men.

Disorders like multiple sclerosis, spina bifida, Parkinson's disease, strokes, and spinal cord injury can all interfere with nerve function of the bladder.

During urination, detrusor muscles in the wall of the bladder contract, forcing urine out of the bladder and into the urethra. At the same time, sphincter muscles surrounding the urethra relax, letting urine pass out of the body. Incontinence will occur if the bladder muscles suddenly contract or muscles surrounding the urethra suddenly relax.

Types of incontinence

- ❖ Stress incontinence: As a result of chronic cough, weight lifting, and strenuous exercises.
- ❖ Urge incontinence: Due to sudden urge for no specific reason, there is voiding of urine as in UTI.
- ❖ Overflow incontinence: Due to bladder pouring out urine even after their normal discharge, often termed dribbling of urine. This occurs in uterine prolapsed, after multiple pregnancies etc.
- ❖ Structural incontinence: Rarely, structural problems can cause incontinence.
- ❖ Functional incontinence: It happens when there is a need to go to a rest room when one feels the urge or need, but

one is physically unable to make it to the toilet for multiple reasons such as poor mobility, anger, depression, poor eye sight, poor dexterity, or even unable to find a washroom during a journey.

- Bedwetting is episodic UI while asleep. It is normal in young children.
- Transient incontinence is a temporary version of incontinence. It can be triggered by medications, adrenal insufficiency, mental impairment, restricted mobility, and stool impaction (severe constipation) which can push against the urinary tract and obstruct outflow.
- Giggle incontinence is an involuntary response to laughter. It usually affects children.

Training

Regular exercises and yogic postures to strengthen the pelvic floor muscles will prevent incontinence due to laxed muscles and ligaments.

Holistic approach

Homeopathy

The main aim in giving homeopathic medicines is to strengthen the muscles of the bladder which are responsible for the voiding. The objective is to form a balance between the intra-abdominal pressure, urinary bladder pressure, and urethral pressure.

The cause and type of urinary incontinence will differentiate the homeopathic medicines and their approach as well. For example, giggle incontinence is more common in children between 5–7 years of age, and it will subside by its own as age advances. In case of structural incontinence the causative factor is important; if it is vesico vaginal fistula then the line of management of dealing with the incontinence is different as it requires deep acting remedies most of the time.

Causticum 200, Squilla 200, Pulsatilla 200, and Nux Vom 200 are very good to cure incontinence.

Naturopathy

General treatments to strengthen the bladder and pelvic floor muscles like hip baths, spinal baths, abdomen compress, and packs can be done. Pelvic floor exercises are suggested to regain the strength of the pelvic muscles.

Ayurveda

Depending on the causative factor, the line of treatment will differ. Internal medications are given to eliminate infections, if any, and also to strengthen the bladder. Murivenna Pichu helps strengthen the bladder and pelvic floor muscles. Apart from this, general treatments for rejuvenation help. In case of multiple sclerosis, medicines to strengthen the nerves are prescribed.

CERVICITIS

Cervicitis, a common infection of the lower genital tract, is the inflammation of the cervix (this is the neck and outlet of a woman's uterus). Inflammation may be caused by infection from certain sexually-transmitted diseases (STDs) or by injury to the cervix from a foreign object inserted in the vagina, from birth control devices such as the cervical cap or a diaphragm, or by cancer. If untreated, cervicitis may lead to pelvic inflammatory disease, infertility, ectopic pregnancy, chronic pelvic pain, spontaneous abortion, cervical cancer, or other complications during the delivery of a baby. Risk factors for the development of cervicitis include starting intercourse at an early age, high-risk sexual behaviours, a history of sexually-transmitted diseases, and having multiple sex partners.

Causes

- ❖ Sexually-transmitted infections such as gonorrhoea, chlamydia, and trichomoniasis.
- ❖ Injury to the area.
- ❖ Chemical reactions.
- ❖ Latex allergy from contraceptive use.
- ❖ Insertion of foreign and unsanitized objects into the vaginal canal.
- ❖ Sperm allergy.
- ❖ Unsafe sexual practices.
- ❖ Risky sexual behaviour such as having multiple sexual partners. HIV, infection with the herpes virus (genital herpes), and human papillomavirus (HPV, genital warts) can cause cervicitis.

Symptoms

- ❖ Abnormal vaginal discharge that has foul odour.
- ❖ Greyish, whitish, or yellowish discharge.
- ❖ Abnormal vaginal bleeding.
- ❖ Pelvic, abdominal, and vaginal pain.
- ❖ Burning sensation when urinating.
- ❖ Vaginal pain during sexual intercourse.
- ❖ Swollen cervix.

Prevention

Females suffering from cervical inflammation should prevent the use of chemicals like douches and deodorant tampons.

Spermicidal contraceptives or condoms should be used to prevent sexually-transmitted diseases.

Resorting to a single sexual partner and decent hygiene should be maintained to prevent cervical inflammation. This includes washing after sexual intercourse, urinating after intercourse etc.

Hormonal therapy may be used in women who have reached menopause, but only if absolutely necessary.

Holistic approach

Simple cervicitis usually heals with treatment if the cause is found and relevant treatments are done. This would include treatments from ayurveda, naturopathy, and homeopathic internal medications. Simple lifestyle changes help as well.

Homeopathic medicines treat the underlying cause and increase the power of the immune system to overthrow the infection.

Naturopathy

Naturopathic vaginal douches with neem water, sitz baths, and hip baths are used to treat acute infections.

Ayurveda

Treatments to reduce inflammation and to maintain the pH of the mucosa are given like herbal douches, herbal hip bath, and herbal applications help. Internal medications are also helpful.

Urinary Tract Infection

Urinary tract infection is very common, especially in the fertile age group and post menopause.

Causes

The reasons for its occurrence vary. It could spread from an infected toilet, or it could be the result of antibiotic intake, reduced water intake, as a symptom of renal stones, cystic irritation post coitus etc. Post menopause, its occurrence is frequent due to hormonal changes causing dryness or change in the microbial flora lining the mucosa.

Sometimes it could also be due to bladder or renal infections. In diabetics too, frequent UTI could occur.

Common Symptoms

The symptoms of UTI vary. It could just be increased frequency of urination or present with stronger symptoms such as a burning sensation, severe pain in the pubic region radiating to the entire pelvic region, or one could get high fever with chills. Some cases are accompanied by vomiting and there could be blood in the urine, with or without pus.

If these symptoms are left untreated, they could ascend into the kidneys, causing infection.

Prevention

- Drink lots of water, at least 10–12 glasses per day.
- Take precautions while using public toilets, like wiping the toilet seat with antiseptic wipes.
- Maintain general hygiene, like washing up after every urination and defecation.
- Avoid using soap too much. It causes dryness in the area.
- Avoid green chillies and highly spicy food.

Holistic approach

Holistic approach in UTIs is to elicit the causative factor. This is done through an elaborate history taking, where stress and other emotions are also considered.

Since lifestyle is given importance, any changes made would be advised accordingly.

As per the cause, treatments, internal medications, easy to follow dietary tips, simple yoga etc. are advised. Specific treatments and exercises to strengthen the bladder are taught.

Further occurrence is prevented and the changes or damages done due to the previous infections are reversed.

Homeopathy

Cantharis can be taken frequently for urinary tract infection. Berberis Vulgaris Q in water is a good remedy for the burning and pain during urination. Sarasaparilla can be used when there is burning in urethra after urination. Nux Vom is also a good remedy for pain and burning with urination especially with ineffectual desire for urination. Recurrent UTIs need to be evaluated by a homeopathic doctor and appropriate constitutional remedies can completely cure the complaint.

Naturopathy

- Drinking alkaline juices and drinks help prevent and get rid of the symptoms of UTI.
- Ash gourd or white pumpkin juice, tender coconut water mixed with finely powdered cardamom, cranberry juice, juice of plantain stem, barley water, and drinking plenty of plain water relieves the symptoms.
- Sitting in a tub of cold water, immersing between ribs and thighs helps.
- Applying cold mud or a wet pack on the lower abdomen reduces burning and pain.
- For itching, washing the genital region with neem water helps.
- If the UTI is because of deranged pH of the mucosal lining, washing with curd or buttermilk helps too.

- Intake of curd and buttermilk should be increased.
- Applying castor oil to the lower abdomen can ease the discomfort that comes with UTI.

Ayurveda

- Water boiled with Gokshura (Tribulus Terrastris) and Punarnava (Borhevia Diffusa) helps to flush out toxins.
- Arrow root water helps to relieve the pain and burning sensation.
- Water boiled with a group of herbs called Nalpamara is used to wash the area, in order to alter the pH.
- To give the effect of antibiotics, Brihatyadi Kashayam and Chandra Prabha Gulika is helpful as they control infection.
- To clear the post-voidal urine, Vastyamayandakagritham is given.

Itching in the Vagina and Fungal Infection

Vaginal itching and fungal infections occur due to various reasons. It could be acquired due to the altered pH in the mucosa, as a reaction to, or as a result of, some medications, post menstruation etc. It is usually acquired as a result of toilet sharing, wearing damp clothes, and tight undergarments.

Prevention

- Take precautions while using public toilets, like wiping the toilet seat with antiseptic wipes.
- Maintain general hygiene like washing up after every urination and defecation.
- Special care to be taken during menstruation like changing the napkins regularly and washing the area frequently.
- Remove excess pubic hair regularly through safe methods, followed by antiseptic measures.

- Avoid using soap too much. It causes dryness in the area.
- Wash undergarments thoroughly with hot water and mild detergent, sun dry, and iron them before reusing.
- Wear only cotton under garments, as they let in air, where as the synthetic ones prevent air circulation and trap moisture.

Holistic approach

The approach is to bring about lifestyle changes including hygiene, diet, and exercises. Medications and treatments as per the individual condition are prescribed.

Homeopathy

Kreosotum can be taken when there is thick white offensive discharge, combined with burning and pain in the vagina. Caladium is a good remedy when there is severe itching in vagina in young girls. Homeopathic constitutional remedies like Pulsatilla, Nitric acid, Sepia are also good in treating vaginal infection and white discharges.

Naturopathy

- Washing with neem decoction helps to curb infection.
- Water boiled with turmeric and cooled to room temperature is also helpful.
- Sitting in a tub filled with water boiled with neem and turmeric for 20 minutes twice a day helps too.
- Washing the genitalia with thin sour buttermilk helps the condition.

Ayurveda

- Washing with decoctions of triphala, Nalpamara etc. helps to reduce the itching and burning sensation.
- Applications like Satadhouta Gritham, Mahatikta Gritham will help reduce dryness and itching.

PCOS

Polycystic ovarian syndrome (PCOS) is a problem in which a woman's hormones are out of balance. It can cause problems with your periods and make it difficult to get pregnant. PCOS may also cause unwanted changes in the way you look. If it is not treated, it can lead to serious health problems over time.

Causes

It is one of the most common female endocrine disorders. PCOS is a complex, heterogeneous disorder of uncertain etiology, but there is strong evidence that it can, to a large degree, be classified as a genetic disease.

Hormones are chemical messengers that trigger many different processes, including growth and energy production. Often, the job of one hormone is to signal the release of another hormone. In PCOS the hormones get out of balance. One hormone change triggers another, which changes another.

PCOS produces symptoms in approximately 5 percent to 10 percent of women of reproductive age (12–45 years). It is thought to be one of the leading causes of female sub-fertility, and is the most frequent endocrine problem in women in this age bracket.

Common symptoms

The principal features are anovulation (absence of ovulation) resulting in irregular menstruation (amenorrhoea), ovulation-related infertility, and polycystic ovaries; excessive amounts or effects of androgenic (masculinizing) hormones, resulting in acne and hirsutism and insulin resistance, often associated with obesity, Type-2 diabetes, and high cholesterol levels. The symptoms and severity of the syndrome vary greatly among affected women.

Symptoms

Symptoms tend to be mild at first. You may have only a few symptoms or a lot of them. The most common symptoms are:

- Acne.
- Weight gain and trouble losing weight.
- Extra hair on the face and body. Often women get thicker and darker facial hair and more hair on the chest, belly, and back.
- Thinning hair on the scalp.
- Irregular periods. Often women with PCOS have fewer than nine periods a year. Some women have no periods. Others have very heavy bleeding.
- Fertility problems. Many women who have PCOS have trouble getting pregnant.
- Depression.
- Most women with PCOS grow many small cysts on their ovaries. That is why it is called polycystic ovarian syndrome. The cysts are not harmful but lead to hormone imbalances.
- Menstrual disorders, oligomenorrhoea (few menstrual periods), or amenorrhoea (no menstrual periods), and other types of menstrual disorders may also occur.
- Infertility results directly from chronic anovulation (lack of ovulation).
- High levels of male hormones.
- The most common signs are acne and acanthosis nigricans (darkened skin patches in skin creases, especially on the back of the neck).
- Hirsutism, and it may produce hypermenorrhoea (very frequent menstrual periods) or other symptoms.
- Approximately three-quarters of patients with PCOS have evidence of hyperandrogenemia.
- Metabolic syndrome: This appears as a tendency towards central obesity and other symptoms associated with

insulin resistance. Serum insulin, insulin resistance, and homocysteine levels are higher in women with PCOS.

Prevention

Where PCOS is associated with obesity, successful weight loss is the most effective method of restoring normal ovulation/menstruation, but many women find it very difficult to achieve and sustain significant weight loss.

Low carbohydrate diets and sustained regular exercise may help. Some experts recommend a low GI (Glycemic Index) Diet in which a significant part of total carbohydrates are obtained from fruit, vegetables, and whole grain sources.

Vitamin-D deficiency may play some role in the development of the metabolic syndrome, so treatment of any such deficiency is indicated. A sequence of exercises targeting the pelvic muscles and organs has shown some success in inducing menstruation and ovulation.

Holistic approach

A holistic approach analyzes the cause for the disease. Lifestyle changes, diet, and exercise helps a lot in regularizing the hormones, helps in losing weight, and also regularize the periods. Ayurvedic and homeopathic internal medications help to enhance the changes in the body, especially to tone and strengthen the reproductive system. Counselling helps the person to overcome fears, inhibitions and complexes if any. Specific treatments help in weight loss and to tone the uterus and the ovaries.

Homeopathy

- Causative factor being genetic in a few cases, it is difficult to completely cure the PCOS. But symptomatic treatment can be planned.

- Homeopathy has good remedies to regularize the menstrual cycles, and cysts are treatable.
- By regularizing hormone levels, ovulation is stimulated and chances of fertility are improved.
- Symptomatic treatments can also be planned for PCOS patients depending on the symptoms. Constitutional medicines like Nat Mur, Nat Carb, Calc Carb, Puls, Sepia, Silica Thuja, Kali Carb are selected on an individual basis depending on the case analysis.
- Acute medicines—Sabina, Viburnum Op, Pulsatila, Calc Flour Aur Mur Nat, Cimcifuga, Kreosote, Thalaspi, Theocinum, Caulophylum, and Fraxinus Americana.
- These acute medicines are selected according to the symptoms.

Naturopathy

Treatments such as hip bath, acupuncture, abdomen compress and T-packs are specific for PCOS. Yogic postures like Baradwajasana, Ushtrasana, Vakrasana, Ardha Matsyendrasana, and Yoga Mudrasana help to strengthen the uterine muscles and the ovaries. Pranayama such as Kapalabhati, Ujjayi, and Brahmari too help the reproductive system.

Ayurveda

Panchakarma treatments help to cleanse the ovaries and uterus, to stabilize the hormones, and to control the weight gain. Internal medications to reduce the cysts and to tone the functions of uterus and ovaries help. It also helps to control associated symptoms like hair fall and dry skin.

Painful Sex (Dyspareunia)

Painful intercourse can occur for a variety of reasons, ranging from structural problems to psychological concerns. Many women experience painful intercourse at some point in their lives.

The medical term for painful intercourse is dyspareunia. Pain during or after sexual intercourse is also known as dyspareunia.

Although this problem can affect men, it is more common in women.

Women with dyspareunia may have pain in the vagina, clitoris or labia, which is defined as persistent or recurrent genital pain that occurs just before, during or after intercourse. Talk to your doctor if you're experiencing painful intercourse. Treatments focus on the underlying cause, and can help eliminate or reduce this common problem.

Causes

There are numerous causes of dyspareunia, many of which are treatable.

- Physical causes of painful intercourse tend to differ, depending on whether the pain occurs at entry or with deep thrusting.
- Emotional factors can be associated with many types of painful intercourse.
- Insufficient lubrication is also commonly caused by a drop in estrogen levels after menopause, after childbirth or during breastfeeding. In addition, certain medications are known to inhibit desire or arousal, which can decrease lubrication and make sex painful. These include antidepressants, high blood pressure medications, sedatives, antihistamines, and certain birth control pills.

- Atrophic Vaginitis, a common condition causing thinning of the vaginal lining in postmenopausal women.
- An allergic reaction to clothing, spermicides, or douches.
- Endometriosis, an often painful condition in which tissue from the uterine lining migrates and grows abnormally inside the pelvis.
- Inflammation of the area surrounding the vaginal opening, called Vulvar Vestibulitis.
- Skin diseases, such as Lichen Planus and Lichen Sclerosis, affecting the vaginal area.
- Urinary tract infections,vaginal yeast infections, or sexually-transmitted diseases.
- Psychological trauma, often stemming from a history of sexual abuse or trauma.
- Injury or irritation from an accident, pelvic surgery, female circumcision, episiotomy, or a congenital abnormality.
- An infection in your genital area or urinary tract can also cause painful intercourse. Eczema or other skin problems in your genital area can also be the problem.
- Emotions are deeply intertwined with sexual activity and may play a role in any type of sexual pain. Emotional factors include:
    - Psychological problems: Anxiety, depression, concerns about your physical appearance, fear of intimacy or relationship problems can contribute to a low level of arousal and a resulting discomfort or pain.
    - Stress: Your pelvic floor muscles tend to tighten in response to stress in your life. This can contribute to pain during intercourse.

Symptoms

Women with dyspareunia may feel superficial pain at the entrance of the vagina, or deeper pain during penetration or thrusting of the penis.

Some women also may experience severe tightening of the vaginal muscles during penetration, a condition called Vaginismus.

Prevention

Timely help should be sought to prevent damage to one's emotional self and marital harmony.

If dyspareunia occurs after pregnancy, you need to wait at least 6 weeks after childbirth and gentle and safe sex is advisable after 6 weeks.

If pain is mild to moderate, simple home care is enough to get rid from dyspareunia.

If dyspareunia is due to vaginal dryness, then apply water based lubricants or natural lubricants.

To avoid infection, urinate after sexual intercourse.

To decrease your risk of yeast infection, avoid tight clothing, wear cotton underpants, and practice good hygiene.

Change your underclothes after prolonged sweating. Bathe or shower daily, and change into dry clothing promptly after swimming.

Holistic approach

Homeopathy

Depending on the cause of dyspareunia, remedies are administered.

- Dryness of vagina: Nat Mur, Sepia Platina.
- Vaginal infection: Borax, Kreosote.
- Cystitis due to dyspereunia: Cantharis, Berberis, Sepia, Caust.
- Injury: Arnica, Rhus Tox, Staphy.

Naturopathy

Packs like T-pack and abdomen compresses, hip baths, and

sitz baths help overcome the tightness of the pelvic muscles.

A relaxing full immersion bath with few drops of essential oils of rose, lavender, or jasmine helps relax the muscles and the mind and prevent pain.

Ayurveda

Treatments to de-stress, maintain the hormones and to remove the vaginal dryness through lubrication with medications such as Satadhauta Gritham will be done.

Heavy Menstruation

Heavy menstrual bleeding is medically called as menorrhagia.

The usual length of menstrual bleeding is 4–6 days. The usual amount of blood loss per period is 10 to 35 ml. Each soaked normal-sized tampon or pad holds a teaspoon (5 ml) of blood. That means it is normal to soak 1–7 normal-sized pads or tampons (sanitary products) in a whole period.

Officially, flow of more than 80 ml (or 16 soaked sanitary products) per menstrual period is considered menorrhagia.

In summary, very heavy menstrual bleeding relates to soaking 12 or more regular sanitary products in one period. About 25 percent of women in early perimenopause, some teens, and a few women of other ages experience this type of bleeding.

It is an abnormally heavy and prolonged menstrual period at regular intervals. Menorrhagia can be caused by abnormal blood clotting, disruption of normal hormonal regulation of periods, or disorders of the endometrial lining of the uterus. Depending upon the cause, it may be associated with abnormally painful periods.

Causes

- Heavy flow is most common in the teens and in perimenopause—both are times of the lifecycle when estrogen levels tend to be higher and progesterone levels to be lower.
- Progesterone is produced by the ovaries after ovulation. However, even though you may be having regular periods, it doesn't mean you are ovulating!
- The lining of the uterus or endometrium sheds during a period. Estrogen's job is to make the endometrium thicker and more likely to shed during menses.
- And progesterone makes it thinner. Therefore it is likely that heavy flow is caused by too much estrogen and too little progesterone.
- Most common causes include blood disorder or stress-related disorders.

Prevention

- Keep a record—Make a careful record of your flow for a cycle or two. Note—if the flow is so heavy that you start to feel faint or dizzy when you stand up, consult with your doctor.
- Treat blood loss with extra fluid and salt—When you feel dizzy or your heart starts pounding after you get up from lying down, it shows that the amount of blood volume in your system is too low. To help that, drink more liquids and increase the salty fluids you drink such as tomato or other vegetable juices or salty broths. You will likely need at least 4–6 cups (1-1.5 litre) of extra liquid on those days.
- Take iron to replace what is lost with heavy bleeding—You can also increase the iron you get from foods. Red meat, liver, egg yolks, deep green vegetables, and dry fruits like raisins and prunes are good sources of iron.

Holistic approach

We look at the over all picture, take into account various contributing factors like heredity, stress, exercise, nutrition, and functional variations. Based on these, internal medications from ayurveda and homeopathy along with external treatments are given. This helps in long term regularization. Since these do not have any synthetic hormones, it actually regulates the hormone secretions to bring about long-term effects.

Acupuncture is also included to strengthen the uterus and the ovaries, to de-stress and regularize hormones.

Homeopathy

Heavy bleeding is due to hormone imbalance and is a symptom of PCOS. Constitutional treatment is planned and acute medicines are given to immediately subside the menstrual flow. Thebest homeopathic medicines which are frequently used are Sabina, Mellifolium, Thalaspi, Puls, China, Fraxinus American, Viburnum Op, and Nux Vom.

Naturopathy

The reasons being either hormonal or organ related, the approach is through external treatments, diet, and exercises.

Treatments for strengthening the pelvic organs like hipbaths, sitz baths, abdomen compresses, and T-packs are done regularly. Diet should include a lot of iron and calcium and rich sources like leafy vegetables, ragi, skim-milk products, dry fruits like dates, black raisins, and prunes.

Ayurveda

Medication for physical or structural changes, stress and treatments like herbal hip baths, Abhyanga, and Sirodhara are advised.

Medications like Muslikadiradi Kashayam, Sukumara Kashayam, and Pusyanuga Choornam are helpful.

Yoga

Yogic asanas like Baddha Konasana, Vakrasana, Ardha Matsyendrasana, Yoga Mudrasana, Suryanamaskar along with meditation and pranayamas like Kapalabhati, Nadi Shodhana, and Brahmari help to regularize the menstruation.

Absent Menstruation

Absent menses is also called as amenorrhoea. It is generally of two kinds. The first is primary amenorrhoea i.e. when a girl has not yet started her monthly periods but she has gone through other normal changes that occur during puberty like breast development, pubic hair etc. The girls are generally older than 15 years. The second kind is secondary amenorrhoea which occurs when a woman who has been having normal menstrual cycles stops getting her periods for 6 or more months. It occurs in absence of pregnancy and lactation, suppression of normal cycle with hormonal contraceptive pills or menopause.

Causes

Most girls begin menstruating between ages 9 and 18, with an average around 12-years old.

- Primary amenorrhoea typically occurs when a girl is older than 15, if she has undergone other normal changes that occur during puberty.
- Primary amenorrhoea may occur with or without other signs of puberty.
- Being born with poorly formed genital or pelvic organs (missing uterus or vagina, vaginal septum, cervical stenosis,

or imperforate hymen) can lead to primary amenorrhoea.

❖ Hormones play a big role in a woman's menstrual cycle. Hormone problems can occur when:
  - Changes occur to the parts of the brain where hormones that help manage the menstrual cycle are produced.
  - The ovaries are not working correctly, maybe due to genetic defects.
  - Infections that occur in the womb or after birth.
  - Other birth defects.
  - Tumours.

Other causes include:

❖ Brain (pituitary) tumours.
❖ Polycystic ovarian syndrome.
❖ Premature ovarian failure.
❖ Thyroid dysfunction.
❖ Chemotherapy drugs for cancer.

Factors that can disrupt normal menstruation and cause secondary ammenorrhoea include:

❖ Drastic weight loss.
❖ Eating disorders.
❖ Pregnancy.
❖ Stress and anxiety.
❖ Significant weight gain or obesity.
❖ Hormonal imbalance (such as with polycystic ovarian syndrome).
❖ Endocrine disorders such as thyroid disease or pituitary disease/tumour.

Common symptoms

Amenorrhoea is a symptom of an underlying disorder rather than a condition in itself. Additional symptoms may be present depending on the associated condition. Galactorrhoea (breasts produce milk in a woman who is not pregnant or breastfeeding), headaches, hirsutism may be caused by excess androgen (a hormone that encourages development of male sex characteristics). Vaginal dryness, hot flashes, night sweats or disordered sleep may be a sign of ovarian insufficiency or premature ovarian failure. Noticeable weight gain or weight loss may be present. Excessive anxiety may be present in women with associated psychiatric abnormalities, acne, cyclic pain without bleeding are also symptoms.

Prevention

- Keep monitoring girls at pubertal age. If there is a delayed menstrual cycle or underdeveloped secondary sex hormones, immediately consult your gynaecologist.
- If there is a family history of puberty at 15 or 16 years, then you can wait till that period to get a normal flow.
- In secondary amenorrhoea a lot of hormonal medicines, or contraceptive pills can lead to an absence of flow, so it's better to avoid most of them. Maintain your weight levels.
- Take nutritious food.
- Get regular checks done with hormonal tests and scans, which can give you theproper information regarding your reproductive system.

Holistic approach

The approach segregates the cause as to genetic, organ malformation, nutrition, and hormonal. Treatments and internal medications are then prescribed. This would mainly mean to detoxify the system, rejuvenate, and stimulate better organ function. Counselling helps to improve self-confidence and ensure better mental perspective.

The internal medications are herbal in origin and do not contain any steroids or hormones. They only help the proper functioning of the internal organs.

Homeopathy
Primary menstrual absence is due to under developed growth hormones. Homeopathic remedies successfully used in this condition are Thyroidinum, Medorrhenum Thuja, Sepia, and Iodum.

Secondary menstrual absence is due to improper secretion of hormones and other contributing factors and successfully used medicines are Nat Carb, Calc Carb, Thuja Puls, Cimcifuga, Graphitis, Nat Mur.

Naturopathy
The approach is the same as in any other menstrual disorder. Treatments to strengthen the reproductive system like hip baths, packs and compresses, proper nutrition, and dietary advice are provided. Acupuncture also helps in stimulating the organ function. Special yogic techniques like Baddha Konasana, Yogamudrasana, Vakrasana, and Suryanamskars are given along with pranayamas and meditation.

Ayurveda
De-stress and detoxification treatments like Abhyanga, Sirodhara, Nasya, and Vasti should be done. These procedures could be done with herbs that help tone the uterus.

Herbal hip baths help. Sukumaram Kashayam, Lodhradi Kashayam, Rajapravartini Vati, Palasarpis, and Ashoka Gritham are all used internally.

Chewing sesame seeds with palm jaggery helps as a home remedy.

Menstrual Cramps

Menstrual cramps occur mostly in the abdomen, though some women tend to feel them on the lower back, inner thighs, or calves. This occurs due to the hormonal changes during menstruation, and also as a result of the loss of electrolytes through menstrual blood. The abdominal cramping is found to be more on consumption of gas producing food such as the high protein food like lentils, beans, and fermented food.

Prevention

- Warm castor oil application around the navel and lower abdomen.
- A hot compress to the abdomen, inner thighs, and lower back.
- A glass of hot water with a teaspoon of ghee mixed in.
- A hot infusion of fresh ginger with few drops of lime juice added into it.
- Take only light food during the first 2 days of menstruation and a day before the onset.
- Avoid deep fried, heavy food and high protein food like rajma, meat, and soya just before menstruation.

Holistic approach

Homeopathy

Caulophylum 200, Magphos 3x, Colocynth 200, and Vibernum opulus 200 are all prescribed to help relieve menstrual cramps.

Ayurveda

Serrac Asoka, Satavari (Asparagus Racemoses), Aloevera, and Butea Frondosa in various combinations help to strengthen the uterus and the reproductive system and to prevent menstrual cramps.

Herbal hip baths, pichu on the lower abdomen, and Vasti are treatments which help prevent menstrual cramps.

Spotting

Spotting is light bleeding which occurs at a time when the woman's period is not expected. It could be due to various reasons—hormonal or functional. Once the reason is diagnosed, one should go in for proper medical examination to ascertain the cause. Depending on the cause, the correct treatments would be suggested.

Holistic approach

Treatments to strengthen the reproductive system which include various baths, and massages and internal medication to improve uterine muscles and strengthen the reproductive system help in general.

Homeopathy
Pulsatilla 30, Sabena 30, China 200, and Bryonia 200 are prescribed for spotting.

Naturopathy
Abdomen compresses, T-packs, and hip baths are the naturopathic remedies for spotting.

Ayurveda
Asoka (Serraca Asoka), Satavari (Asparagus racemoses), Aloevera, and Butea Frondosa in various combinations help to control spotting. Along with these, herbal hip baths, massages help too.

PMS

Premenstrual syndrome is a symptom complex which accompanies the menstrual cycle. This is seen to show up few days to a week prior to the onset of menstruation. Generally this passes off as the normal menstrual flow set in. The symptoms include aches, pain in the abdomen, back or legs, irritability, sleeplessness, headaches, migraines, food cravings, short temperedness, sadness, depression, stress, water retention, and bowel irregularities. One or few of the above said symptoms are seen generally. The intensity of the symptoms varies from cycle to cycle.

This arises as a result of the hormonal changes occurring with menstruation.

Holistic Approach

Yoga and exercise play a very important role in controlling these symptoms as they take care of the mind and the body. They are more preventive in nature.

Homeopathy

Pulsatilla 200 or 30, Ignatia 200, Natrum Muraticum 1m as constitutional medicines are given in homeopathy to control PMS.

Naturopathy

Naturopathic treatments like the mud baths, steam baths, water jet baths, hip baths, spinal baths, and abdomen compresses help according to the symptoms.

Eating moderately, including fruits and vegetables and lot of fluids help to prevent the symptoms.

Ayurveda

Asoka (Serraca Asoka), Lodhra, Satavari (Asparagus

Racemoses), and Red Sandal are the herbs which would help control PMS.

Dryness of Vagina

Vaginal dryness is a common symptom of vaginal atrophy called Atrophic Vaginitis. The dryness of vagina is because of lack of female hormone (estrogen) production, which causes thinning and inflammation of the vaginal walls.

Dryness of vagina can be seen during and after menopause though it can develop at any age because of lack of lubrication. Vaginal dryness can make intercourse uncomfortable. Most vaginal lubrication consists of clear fluid that seeps through the walls of the blood vessels encircling the vagina. When you're sexually aroused, more blood flows to your pelvic organs, creating more lubricating vaginal fluid. But the hormonal changes of menopause, childbirth, and breastfeeding may disrupt this process.

Causes

The causes of vaginal dryness include:

- Decreased estrogen levels because of childbirth, menopause, breastfeeding, immune disorders, cigarette smoking.
- Medications: Antidepressants, allergy and cold medications, anti-estrogen medications which are used to treat breast cancer.
- Sjogren's syndrome.

Symptoms

Symptoms of vaginal dryness include itching, burning, soreness, pain or light bleeding during sex, urinary frequency or urgency.

Holistic approach

Homeopathy

It is most important that the underlying cause should get treated first. The medicines will be given on the basis of symptoms similarity. Constitutional medicines like Natrum Mur, Sepia, Lycopodium, and Graphitis will be helpful in such conditions.

General rejuvenation and detoxification will establish good blood supply and proper functioning of the glands and its secretions. Ayurveda has good medications both internal and for external application. Even the applicants are medicines which help stimulate the natural lubrication and are not just lubricants themselves.

It is possible to alter the pH of the vaginal mucosa through internal medications and treatments from naturopathy, homeopathy, and ayurveda. Acupuncture too helps in this condition.

Naturopathy

Naturopathic treatments like vaginal douche, T- packs etc help in lubrication and to avoid dryness.

Ayurveda

Ayurvedic treatments like Yoni Pichu and external application of Satadhautagritham and Mahatiktakalepam is helpful.

FAQs Related to Holistic Health

Q: Is holistic medicine anti-allopathy?

A: Holistic medicine is **not** anti-allopathy. Many holistic doctors in the west are highly qualified allopathic doctors who are currently practising holistic and integrated medicine.

Q: Is holistic medicine unscientific?
A: The holistic medical approach is based on science and follows scientific methods.

Q: Does holistic medicine have religious connotations?
A: No. It promotes spirituality in health, but has no direct links to religion.

Q: Can anyone practise the therapies and treatments on themselves?
A: A holistic approach to lifestyle and personal habits can be followed by anyone. However, only a trained therapist under the supervision of a doctor should do the medical treatments and therapies.

Q: Are there adverse reactions to mixing other systems of medicines and allopathic medicines?
A: No. Ayurvedic and homeopathy and allopathic medical treatments can be taken simultaneously without any inter-reaction.

Q: The holistic medical approach is generally perceived as a slow process. Are there any quick-fix methods?
A: The natural healing response will be always slow, as the disease process is also slow.

Q: Are there any side effects to integrated medicine?
A: No, as long as a qualified doctor provides it.

Q: How does a massage affect our mind and body?
A: A massage relaxes, rejuvenates, improves circulation, and detoxifies by eliminating toxins from the lymphatic system.

Seven Steps to Holistic Health

1. Meditation

Meditation has been successfully proven to be the most effective tool for stress relief along with several positive physiological effects. It enhances a person's mind and improves memory and concentration. Sessions timed at a minimum 15–20 minutes daily, atleast 5 times a week are ideal.

2. Diet

It is important to have healthy eating habits, eat on time, and drink plenty of fluids. Each person's eating habits should be based on their ancestorss eating habits and should include high amount of fresh vegetables and fruits. Overeating, fast food and high amounts of sugar, salt, and fat are the causes of a majority of today's illnesses.

3. Exercises

A regular exercise pattern for 30–45 minutes daily will keep anybody healthy. Yoga is the best choice or a combination of yoga for half the week and either walking, swimming, jogging, cycling, or aerobics for the rest would be ideal as well.

4. Work

A healthy working environment, good working timings, and mental satisfaction at work are important. A majority of lifestyle-related conditions are caused by stress from work and unhealthy working hours.

5. Relationships

Good personal and emotional relationships with family members and colleagues are important for a healthy life. These enhance a person's quality of life and be an immune booster.

6. Rest

Regular sleep and rest is very important. The person should feel fresh and energetic after a good nights' rest. Around 7–8 hours of sleep and rising early everyday is ideal.

7. Play and Holidays

Playing games and spending time together with friends and family, watching movies, going for holidays on a weekend break or spending time for personal hobbies are important for enhancing health as well.

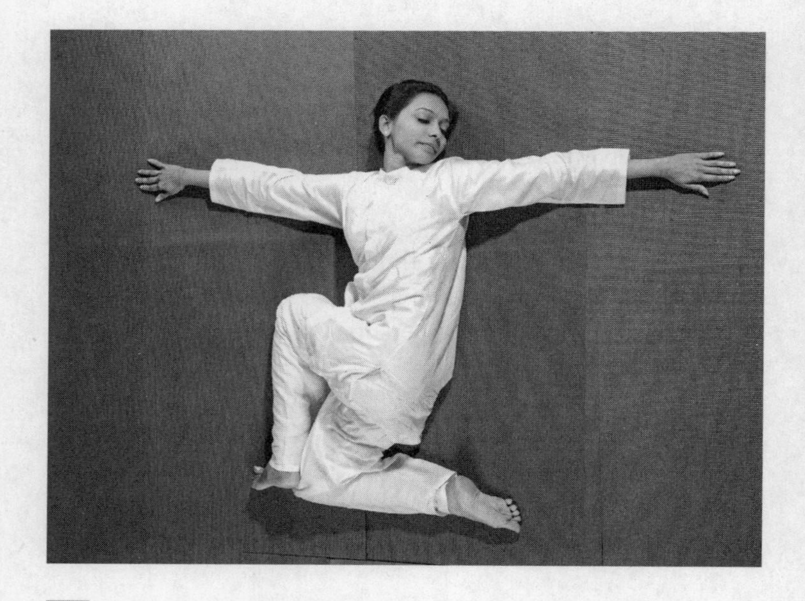

Makarabhyasa (lumbar stretch)

- Lay on the back with the knees bent and feet placed on the ground.
- Extend the arms sideways at the shoulder level.
- Place the right heel on the left knee.
- Inhale and as you exhale, tilt the legs to the left such that the left knee touches the ground on the left side and turn the head to the right.
- Inhale and come back to centre and now place the left heel on the right knee.
- With another exhalation tilt the legs to the right so as to touch the right knee to the ground on the right side and turn the head to the left.
- Repeat it few times and enjoy the relaxation.

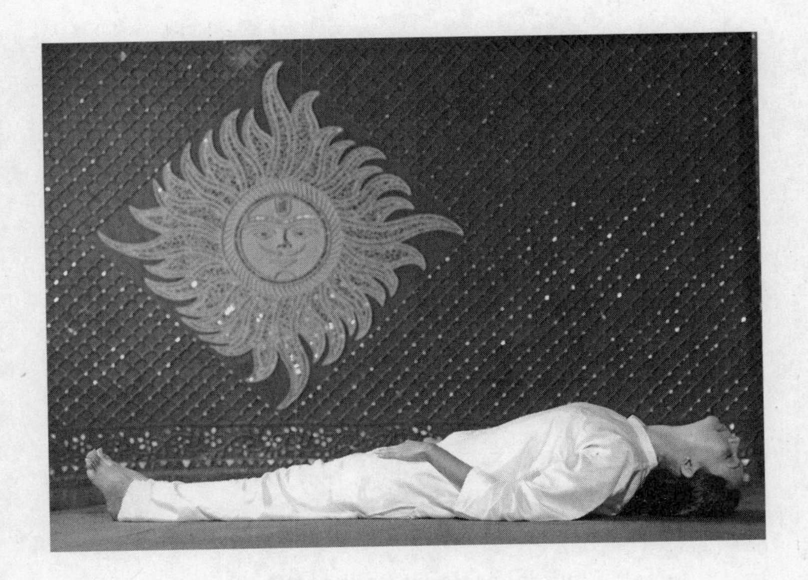

Matsyasana (fish pose)

- Lie on the back, let the legs be together.
- With an inhalation, gently tilt the head and neck backwards such that the crown of the head is touching the ground.
- Lift the shoulders up slightly.
- Now slowly try and cross the legs.
- Place the palms on the respective thigh.
- You can feel the stretch in the neck region.
- With exhalation, slowly straighten the neck and place the head comfortably on the ground.
- Release the legs and keep them apart.
- Let the hands move away from the body.
- Breathe normally while you hold the posture.

Benefits

Matsyasana strengthens the neck and shoulders

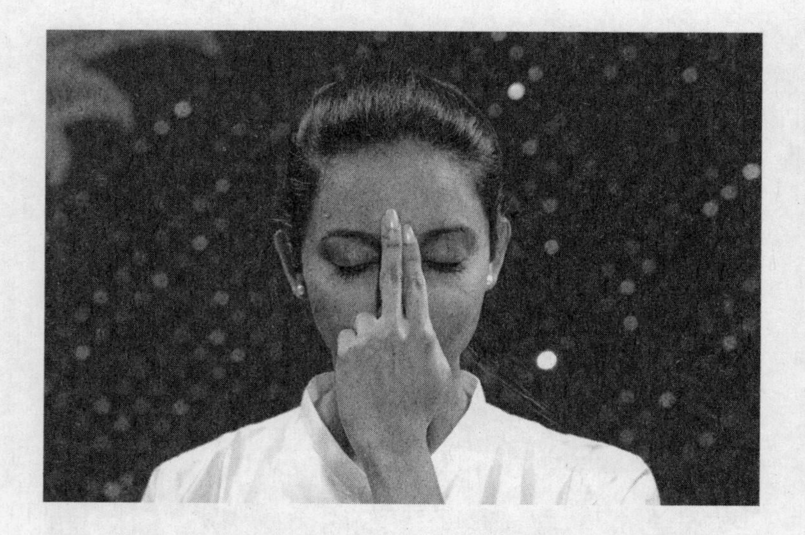

Nadi Shuddhi or Nadi Shodhana Pranayama

Here we have to manipulate the flow of air by exerting a control.

We make use of the right thumb to close the right nostril and the right ring finger to close the left nostril. The index finger and middle finger on the right side can either be bent or placed on the point between the eyebrows.

Now start by inhaling through the left nostril, close it and exhale through the right. Inhale through the right, close it, and exhale through the left. This makes one round of the pranayama. Continue this for a minimum of nine rounds, going up to 27 rounds.

This establishes free flow of air through both the nostrils and also improves the prana in the sushumna nadi.

Note: Generally practicing bandha or locks are adviced, but this needs advanced practice regularly under expert guidance.

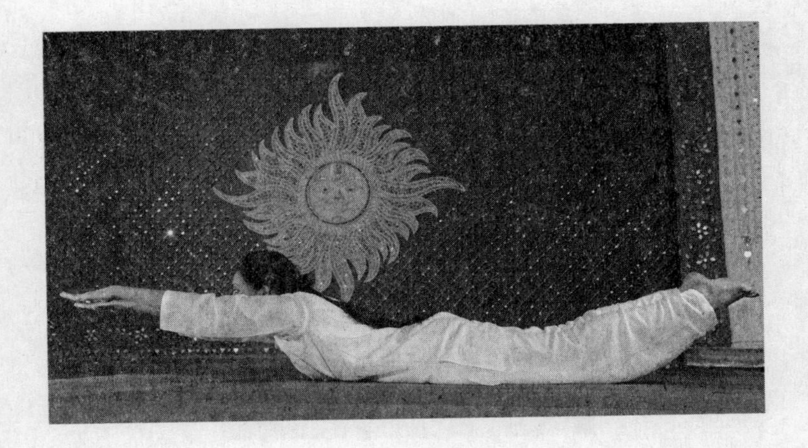

Naukasana (boat pose)

- Lie on the abdomen.
- Bring the legs together, hands by the side of the body, chin touching the ground.
- Now extend the hands to the front of the body.
- Take few deep breaths.
- With an inhalation lift the legs as well as the hands above the ground, balancing on the abdomen.
- Breathe normally and hold the posture comfortably.
- With an exhalation slowly place the legs and arms on the ground and relax.
- Feel the relaxation in the entire back region and the abdominal muscles.

Benefits

This posture improves the tone of the spine • This cuts abdominal fat and strengthens the abdominal recti

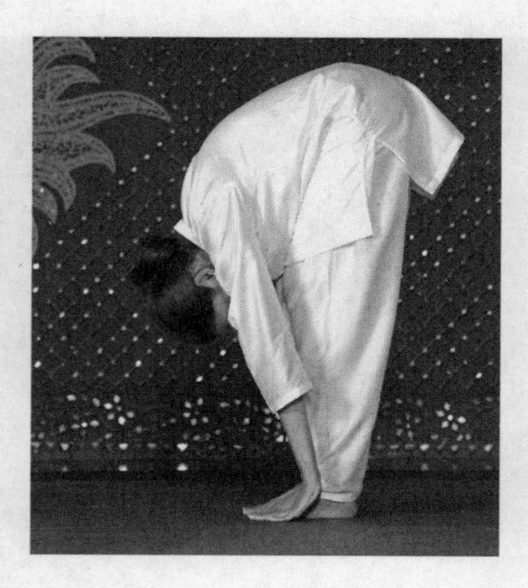

Padahastasana

- Stand straight with the legs together.
- Inhale and raise the arms above the head and slightly bend backwards from the waist.
- With an exhalation, slowly bend forward as much as possible, placing the hands on the legs.
- Continue normal breathing, and with every exhalation, bend down further sliding the hand down, and ultimately placing them on the ground.
- Be aware of the changes you feel in the lower back and stop the movements immediately as you feel the discomfort.
- Do not bend the knees.
- Feel the stretch at the back of the legs.
- Feel the compression in the abdomen.
- Feel the stretch in the lower back.
- With an inhalation, slowly straighten the spine, raising the arms up.
- Exhale and lower the hands to the sides of the body.
- Keep the legs apart and relax.

Benefits

• Padahastasana strengthens the sciatic nerves, tones the muscles and ligaments of the legs • It strengthens the digestive system. • It improves the circulation to the head and neck region

Caution: Please do not practice it when the blood pressure is high. It should also be avoided in cases of slip disc, acute back pain and sciatica.

CHAPTER SIX

Pregnancy and Childbirth

PREGNANCY

A FEMALE BODY IS DESIGNED, SINCE ITS DEVELOPMENTAL stage, from the fusion of ovum and sperm (embryo stage), to help in the conception of or to bear children.

At puberty, menstruation starts, generally between the age of 11 and 14. This is the indication that ovulation has started and the woman is ready to bear children. Menstruation is a process to expel the unfertilized egg from the uterus, and thereby pave way for the next ovulation. Ovulation is the process of the egg maturation and its release into the uterus.

The female reproductive system consists of two ovaries. They are small rounded structures containing millions of eggs. One matured egg is released during each ovulatory cycle. Ovaries take turns, releasing an egg during alternate cycles. The egg or ovum is transported to the uterus through tubes connecting the ovaries to the uterus, called the fallopian tubes.

The matured ovum is received by the uterus with all its preparations, creating a good safe bed, and good blood supply.

The ovum remains active in the uterus for a few days after which it is thrown out along with other tissues and blood as menstrual secretion.

When the ovum is active in the uterus, fertilization could take place. A healthy sperm makes way to the uterus through the vaginal canal and fuses with the ovum, resulting in the formation of a healthy embryo. Following the fusion, cell division occurs, slowly growing into a foetus over a period of 9 months and 7 days (36 weeks).

This period is called pregnancy. The period of pregnancy is calculated from the date of the last menstrual period (LMP). It's the day of onset of the last menstruation. From that day, 9 months and 7 days are added to get the expected date of delivery (EDD). Though this is the date expected, it could always be few days later or before.

A child born anytime before 34 weeks is considered premature. If needed, the child is incubated to provide the uterine atmosphere, to help its growth.

If the delivery is delayed (37 weeks), then the labour is induced through various ways.

Pregnancy and childbirth are important events in a female's life. One should be physically and mentally prepared for these events. One should not conceive by accident; even if it happens, one should immediately start to weave healthy, happy, and good thoughts about the offspring. This helps in the healthy growth of the foetus.

Physically, you should take good care of youself from hygiene to good nutrition to exercise. One should also give proper time for rest and relaxation.

During pregnancy, one is required to sleep for a good 8 hours and also to take a nap post lunch. She should listen to good music and read good books. She should also understand her pregnancy and baby care. She should spend quality time with her husband and be a recipient of his love and care.

She should try and avoid negative thoughts or feelings. Food also plays a major role in a healthy pregnancy and childbirth.

During the initial months of pregnancy, one suffers from

tastelessness, nausea, flatulence, and constipation. During this time it's better to take food in small quantities and at regular intervals. Fruit juices, tender coconut, buttermilk with salt, thin vegetable soups, and rice soups are healthy. Dry food like biscuits, crackers, toast, and rusk can be eaten as they reduce nausea. She should not stop eating food properly, just to avoid the fear of throwing up.

Generally after the initial 3–4 months (1st trimester), these symptoms subside. Now, food intake should be closely monitored. From now on, one will also start gaining weight, with the increasing size of the foetus. The foetus absorbs a lot of nutrition from the mother. Hence the food the mother takes should include all types of nutrients like carbohydrates, proteins, fat, vitamins, minerals, and trace elements.

There could be a craving for junk food etc. during this period. Try to reduce the intake as much as possible, as this leads to unhealthy weight gain and digestive issues.

Try to eat brown rice, whole grain flour chapattis etc. Take proteins adequately through dal, lentils, beans, nuts, seeds, chicken, egg white, fish, and milk products. One should take at least 2 glasses of milk per day to meet the calcium needs of self and the baby. Ragi, green leafy vegetables especially spinach and drumstick leaves are also high sources of calcium.

Anaemia is one condition seen commonly during pregnancy due to the increased blood supply to the foetus. One needs to improve the intake of iron from leafy vegetables, beetroot, dates, and black raisins.

Fruits and vegetables should be taken in plenty. Liquid intake should also be good, with lot of water, thin juices, and soups.

For proper digestion, and to relieve constipation, water, fruit and vegetables help.

There tends to be increased appetite in some people after the 1st trimester. But uncontrolled eating may lead to increased weight gain. Weight gain of more than 12 kilos throughout pregnancy is not advisable, as it would be reflected on the baby's weight. High birth weight could lead to complicated pregnancies needing caesarian section. It could also continue as childhood obesity.

Exercise is important to have healthy pregnancy and childbirth. Moderate walks for 30 minutes every day are advised. This will ensure proper blood circulation. Lack of circulation could lead to swelling in the feet and ankles and cramping of the calves. One often complains of leg pain. Adequate water, regulated salt intake, and proper exercise helps overcome this issue.

Symptoms of pregnancy

Following conception, several changes become noticeable in females like missed monthly periods, salivation, loss of appetite, vomiting, yearning for sour food, heaviness of the body, fatigue, black pigmentation of the lips and areola, appearance of slight swelling of the feet, and dilatation of the genital passage as pregnancy advances.

There are a few very small, but disturbing symptoms during pregnancy. They are dark rings around the eyes, dark pigmentation on different parts of the body, hair loss, stretch marks, and frequent urination. These result due to the changes in the hormones, the skin getting overly stretched with the change in the body shape and gain in weight, and disturbed sleep. Most of these symptoms are relieved gradually after delivery.

Yoga

Yoga asanas and pranayamas help a lot in begetting a healthy baby. There are asanas specified for each trimester. If these asanas are done with care, under an expert guidance, they can give great results. The asanas mainly aim at improving the strength of pelvic bones, to strengthen the abdominal and pelvic muscles, and to remove the stiffness from the groins. Pranayama helps to keep the mind calm and relaxed. It improves the oxygenation to the cells and tissues and also to the foetus, helping the baby's physical and mental growth.

Relaxation techniques are also advised, to relax the body completely and let go of the tightness and stiffness.

Vajrasana should be practiced throughout the pregnancy until the last trimester. Here one sits on the heels, with legs bent at the knees. Buttocks rest on the heels. This posture relieves flatulence and constipation. One could use cushions to support the knees and buttocks if needed.

Yoga for Pregnancy

Practice breathing exercises and pranayamas twice a day during the entire pregnancy.

1–3 Months (1st trimester)

Asanas: Vajrasana, Tadasana, Ardha Chakrasana, Parswa Chakrasana, Viparitakarini, Bhujangasana, Sethubandhasana, Matsyasana, Trikonasana.
Pranayama: Nadi Shodhana, Brahmari, Ujjayi.
All breathing exercises, meditation, and relaxation techniques.

4–7 Months (2nd trimester)

Asanas: Vajrasana, Tadasana, Ardha Chakrasana, Parswa Chakrasana, Viparitakarini, Matsyasana, Janusirasana.
Pranayama: Nadi Shodhana, Brahmari, Ujjayi.
All breathing exercises, meditation, and relaxation techniques.

Last trimester

Asanas: Tadasana, Sethubandhasana, Baddha Konasana, Parswa Chakrasana, Ardha Chakrasana, Baradwajasana.

Pranayama: Nadi Shodhana, Brahmari, Ujjayi, Seetali, Seetkari, Sadanta.
All breathing exercises, meditation, and relaxation techniques to be practiced more frequently.

Unusual Cravings During Pregnancy

Throughout pregnancy, some women develop intense cravings. Some get it at the onset of pregnancy itself. The cravings could be for certain tastes, flavours, particular food or smells.

The most commonly seen craving is for sour taste. Though there is no harm in taking the food one craves for, anything in excess should be avoided, since it could interfere with the baby's growth. Too much sour and spicy food could give acidity as generally during this period, the mucosal linings are tender.

Some unusual cravings are also reported during pregnancy like craving for mud, lime etc. Old people say these are related to being deficient in iron, calcium etc. Such unusual cravings are called 'pica'. According to the nature of the craving, there are effective homeopathic remedies to take care of them.

However these cravings subside mostly after the 1st trimester.

Holistic approach

A holistic approach provides calm, peaceful, happy, and healthy circumstances to the mother, so that it would be reflected on the offspring. This will make the offspring a holistically healthy individual. So the approach would be to educate the parents about the importance of these aspects and guide them through it. It would include treatments, diet plans, exercise programs, and counselling and also provide insight to post delivery care. Homeopathic medicines are very effective for treating cramps.

Importance of Natural Childbirth

Always remember that pregnancy is not a disease. It is a normal physiological process.The changes or symptoms during pregnancy are only because of the change in hormones. So too much medical interference during pregnanacy is not required. One should go for regular checkups just to keep yourself safe.

These days a lot of hype is given to painless labour etc. and in the process, caesarian sections have become common. Instead of being treated as a medical requirement, c-sections are being opted for, sometimes even before conception. Both the lady and the family think it is a safe tool, as they do not have to go through the difficulties of a normal labour and also the time and date of birth could be chosen.

C-section is a life saving method and was invented only to deal situations that are difficult to manage normally. It has its own side effects. C-section is done under spinal anaesthesia, which sometimes leads to permanent back pain. The abdominal muscles are cut, which weakens these muscles and could later lead to a flabby abdomen. There are also higher chances of getting incisional hernia. Post surgical complications like delayed suture healing, pain, inability to breastfeed the child are all commonly seen.

After a c-section, one takes longer to resume the normal exercises which make it difficult to shed the weight.Varicosity is another complication of a caesarian section.

From the medical faculty too, there is a preferance for c-sections. Some doctors find it convenient to recommend c-sections to the individual. Expecting mothers should watch out for such preferences.

However, other natural and effective methods for painless labour, like underwater deliveries, acupuncture for painless labour, homeopathic and ayurvedic medications, and treatments, yogic management through asnanas, pranayama and meditation are highly recommended.

Care of Pregnant Women

Holistic approach

Pregnant women should be looked after affectionately by their husbands and other family members.

For the prevention of damage to the foetus and for the treatment of a woman's illnesses and regimen (consisting of diet and drugs) is necessary.

During the 8th month, Sukhaprasavada Ghrtam is given to tone the pelvic muscles and enable easy delivery.

Anuvasana Vasti (lubricating enema) with ghee processed with sweet tasting drugs is ideal to remove the clogged faeces from the colon.

Enemas with the decoction of dry Moolaka mixed with a paste of Satapushpa, medicated oil, ghee, and Saintava Lavana are ideal.

Milk boiled with the root of murva- Marcedinia tenacissma to nourish the foetus.

Homeopathy

Medicines like Calcarea Carb, Silicea, Num Vom, and Alumina are adviced.

Naturopathy

Naturopathic remedies include gentle body massages, abdomen packs, and foot baths.

Ayurveda

Rather than considering pregnancy as a mere result of physical act, it should be treated as a ritual in itself. One should get rid of any physical ailments and mental disturbances before getting into the act. Panchakarma done appropriately helps in complete detoxification and helps improve the quality of sperm and ovum.

Generally, techniques like Virechanam, Vasti, Uttara Vasti, if needed, all help in the detoxification and strengthening of the reproductive system.

These treatments should be preceded by Sirodhara to strengthen the mind, to regulate the hormones, and for emotional cleansing; Abhyanga to rejuvenate; Sastikapindaswedam to improve the bone density, strengthen pelvic bones, and muscles and to improve calcium absorption; and Pizhichil in cases of vaginal dryness and painful intercourse.

Treatments should be done for *the couple*, depending on the condition, and not just for an individual.

Nutrition is equally important for the embryo and the mother.

CHILDBIRTH

The onset of labour is marked by tiredness, descent of the womb; heaviness of the lower part of the body; pain in the groin, perineum, waist, abdomen and sides; vaginal discharge with or without blood; loss of desire for food and increased frequency of urination.This is followed by labour pains and flow of clear fluid from the vagina.

General tips for a healthy pregnancy and delivery

- The child should be treated as a part of you, as though he/she is experiencing the same feelings/sensations as you are.
- Listen to beautiful music, read stories, and poetry that is beautiful and elevating to the soul.

- Name your baby, and call and talk to him/her.
- Practice meditation, silence, and listen to nature daily.
- Eat healthy, nutritious food.
- Apply oil daily all over your body, specifically to the pelvic region, abdomen, and thighs to avoid stretch marks and relax the muscles.
- Eliminate unhealthy elements from your life including bad air, bad thoughts, and bad food.
- Fresh ginger, cloves, or cinnamon could be used to relieve morning sickness.
- Practice yoga, breathing exercises, and walking everyday.

Holistic approach

Homeopathy

Homeopathic medicines are safe during pregnancy and childbirth. Ipecac is good for vomiting during pregnancy. Nux Vomica can be taken for constipation and ineffectual urge to pass stools. Nux Vomica is also a good remedy for indigestion. Rhus Tox can be taken for general body pains and joint pains during pregnancy. Belladona can be taken for fevers and headaches. Five Phos is a good medicine for general debility and tiredness.

Caulophyllum can be used for progression of labour and for prolonged labour pains. Chamomilla can be used to ease the labour pains and pain after childbirth. Sabina can be given for retained placenta.

Naturopathy

Warm water baths, affusions, and immersions help to relax the muscles and ease labour pain.

Ayurveda

Following delivery, warm water and herbal decoctions which

pacify Vata should be given. Dhanvantaram Kashayam with few drops of Dhanvantaram 101 added to it should be given twice a day, for a month.

After meals, her abdomen should be gently rubbed with oil. A tight abdominal band should be wound regularly to help the involution of uterus and to strengthen abdominal muscles.

It's a general practice to give Pulinkozhambu mixed in medicated buttermilk to drink, to improve digestion and also as a uterine tonic.

She should take showers with warm water before meals.

Water boiled with Nalpamara, tamarind leaves, turmeric, and leaves of jackfruit tree is ideal for bathing.

This routine should be practiced for 5–7 days, as the mother is very sensitive during this period due to the disturbed dhatus. Her energy is depleted during the delivery due to stress and so special care should be taken on her food habits, cleanliness etc.

In the initial 7 days, only thin gruel gradually getting thicker should be given to her. Only after the 7th day , nourishing food should be gradually started.

Meat should not be introduced before 12 days after delivery. This regimen of controlled food, oleation etc. should continue for 45 days.

Yoga

During childbirth there are no postures specifically though Baddha Konasana would help.

Abortion and Miscarriages

A miscarriage is any pregnancy that ends spontaneously at a stage where the foetus is not able to survive independently.

A miscarriage is medically called spontaneous abortion. Miscarriages occurs in 15–20 percent of pregnancies and occurs before the 20th week of pregnancy. Once a foetal heart function is detected in a pregnancy, the chance of miscarriage is less than 5 percent. It is estimated that half of all fertilized eggs are aborted spontaneously before the woman even knows that she is pregnant.

The cause of miscarriage cannot always be detected. The most common causes of miscarriage in the trimester of pregnancy are chromosomal abnormalities, diabetes, hormonal problems, infections, or congenital abnormalities of the uterus.

Exercise, working, and sexual intercourse do not cause pregnancy loss in uncomplicated pregnancies. If the pregnancy is a high risk one, then the woman is advised to refrain from working and also from having sexual intercourse. Smoking is often associated with miscarriage. Paternal smoking also increases the risk of miscarriage. Other factors like alcohol, caffeine, fever, use of NSAID drugs around the time of embryo implant have also been liked to risk of miscarriage.

Signs of miscarriage are abdominal cramping and vaginal bleeding. Vaginal bleeding during early pregnancy is referred to as threatened abortion.

Abortion can be prevented by early, comprehensive prenatal care. Many miscarriages that are caused by systemic diseases like diabetes, thyroid conditions etc. can be prevented by detecting and treating the disease before pregnancy occurs. Exposure to x-rays, use of drugs and alcohol, and high levels of caffeine should be avoided.

Holistic approach

Homeopathy

Homeopathy offers effective treatments in both prevention and combating the effects of abortion which can be psychological and physical. The selection of the homeopathic remedy will be based upon the theory of individualization by using the holistic approach. The aim of homeopathy is not only to manage abortion/miscarriage but to address its underlying cause and individual susceptibility. For individualized remedy selection and treatments, the patient should consult a qualified homeopathic doctor in person.

Given below are some homeopathic remedies which are helpful in the treatment of abortion/miscarriage:

- **Aconite nap:** Threatened abortion caused due to fear and excitement.
- **Apis mel:** Abortion during the 3rd month of pregnancy.
- **Aletris far:** Habitual abortion resulting due to weakness and anaemia.
- **Chamomilla:** Threatened abortion due to mental excitement.
- **Sabina:** Excellent remedy in cases of abortion in every second or third month, habitual abortion, pain in small of back and genitals, bleeding of dark red blood.
- **Sepia:** Abortion during fifth to seventh month of pregnancy.
- **Caulophyllum:** Habitual abortion due to weakness of uterus.
- **Thyroidinum:** Avoids miscarriage and tendency to premature labor when the cause is not mechanical in its origin. Prevents threatened abortion when there is thyroid dysfunction in females, It helps to control slow oozing from uterus.
- **Trillium pend:** Controls or checks bleeding of abortion.
- **Thlaspi:** Abortion with heavy bleeding.
- **Cimicifuga:** Excellent remedy to prevent habitual abortion/ miscarriage should be given in later months of pregnancy to prevent miscarriage.

Naturopathy

Naturopathy too believes in the role of mind and body for proper conception, growth of the foetus and delivery. Diet plays an important role, and so do exercises. As per the advice of the attending physician, exercises should be incorporated. Yoga asanas and pranayamas and meditation practiced regularly can even improve foetal health. Stress plays a major role in causing abortions. One should engage in beautiful thoughts, listen to good music, and read good books to keep the mind stress free.

Ayurveda

Ayurveda advocates preparation of female and male bodies prior to conception. This is to ensure the fertilization of best quality ovum and sperm. Such fertilization, will ensure proper implantation and prevent abortion. Through treatments prior to conception, body and mind are cleansed and prepared to undergo the changes.

At each month, different medicinal preparations are given to ensure proper growth and development of the foetus.

Swollen Feet

Swelling of the feet and ankles can occur as a result of conditions involving the local extremities as well as systemic conditions (diseases and conditions that affect the entire body). Localized processes such as injuries and infections may lead to a swollen foot and/or ankle only on the involved side. Swelling of the ankle on one side is often a result of sprains or strains. Sometimes diseases that affect the entire body, such as heart disease and kidney or liver failure, can result in excess fluid buildup (edema) that is often concentrated in the legs and feet, leading to swelling not only of the ankles but also of the feet and lower legs. This can also occur with obstruction of the venous system, as may occur with pregnancy and obesity. Diseases of the joints, such as arthritis, can also affect the joints of the ankle and foot, leading to swelling of the involved areas. Treatments for swollen ankles and feet depend on the particular cause.

Causes of swollen feet

Swollen feet could be due to many reasons ranging from musculoskeletal and metabolic to circulatory, dietary and lack of exercises or inadequate water intake.

Daily diet should contain approx. 1800 daily calories and be full of heart-healthy foods such as whole grains and healthy fats. Diet should be high in protein to give the muscles tone and definition. Adding in some exercises focusing on the muscles around the ankles will also help you get a toned and defined ankle region, which will help you get rid of those dreaded swollen feet and ankles.

Holistic approach

Holistic treatments aim at analyzing the cause for the swelling and then addressing it through the various treatment techniques and internal medications.

Treatments include the ones for detoxification, rejuvenation, strengthening the muscles and joints, improving circulation and venous return.

Dietary and exercise modifications prevent the same in future.

Homeopathy

Apis is used for pitting edema of the feet with redness of the affected area. Rhus Tox can be used for swelling of the feet with restlessness of leg. Pulsatilla is a good remedy for swelling of feet due to varicose veins.

Naturopathy

Beneficial treatments in such conditions are reverse massages, arm and foot baths, acupuncture and wet packs for legs. Mud baths and applications, packs, and compresses help too.

Ayurveda

The reasons for swollen feet could be many. Depending on the symptoms and the causes the treatments and internal medications vary.

Yoga

Leg raising asanas are best for swollen feet.

Diet

- Salt free diet is preferred.
- Drinking 8–10 glasses of water, apart from lot of fluids also helps.
- Barley water, juice of plantain pith etc. help get rid of the swelling.

Pelvic Floor Muscles

Pelvic floor muscles are the core muscles which help during labour. The pressure of the enlarging uterus is thrust onto these muscles. Hence they bear the brunt of the entire pregnancy and could get weaker.

Even before pregnancy, these muscles should be made stronger. It's possible to strengthen them only through regular exercises. A set of yogic asanas and techniques like Vajrasana, Baradwajasana, Merudandasana, Baddha Konasana, Parswakonasana, Janusirasana, Gomukhasana, Dhanurasana, Veerbhadrasana, Upavistakonasana, Setubandhasana,

Vyagrasana, and Ashwani Mudra help the strengthening of these muscles.

Lactation

As pregnancy sets in, the reproductive system and the breasts undergo a lot of changes, preparing the woman's body for motherhood. Lactation too is an important aspect of this stage. It is the process secreting milk by the mammary glands (breasts) to provide nutrition, hydration, and immunity to the infant.

Care of the breasts should be started during mid pregnancy itself. Any abnormalities in the breasts like inverted nipples or cracked nipples should be treated. Proper hygiene should be maintained. Breasts should be massaged regularly with olive or coconut oil to maintain suppleness.

Breast milk is superior to any other food as it is sterile and reaches the child directly from the mother at room temperature. There is absolutely no chance of developing any allergy to mother's milk. It also provides passive immunity through the antibodies present.

After the first two days of delivery, the colosrum which is secreted throughout pregnancy gets abundant. It is deep yellow fluid which is very high in protein, vit A, sodium, and chloride. It is lower in carbohydrates, fat, and potassium than breast milk. It is rich in antibodies such as IgA, IgM, IgG, which offer immunity and also have a laxative effect. It is rich in vit-D and hence prevents rickets as well.

A healthy mother secretes 500 ml–800 ml of milk every day. One should remember to drink lot of fluids during lactation.

In the first week, the baby should be fed frequently (every 2–3 hours) and by the end of 1st week, it would be done at a 3–4 hour frequency. The initial feed should be for 5–10 minutes at each breast, to condition the reflexes. Later, feeding should be with one breast completely and only then moving to the other breast. Each breast is fed on alternately.

Night feeds may be required initially to keep the baby hunger free, but gradually this should be reduced and one can start giving just boiled and cooled water at night.

Babies should be completely breast fed till 6 months, after which the frequency can be reduced by replacing other feeds. Breastfeeding could be stopped by 12–18 months.

Inadequate milk secretion could happen as a result of infrequent suckling or due to the suppression of prolactin, the hormone responsible for lactation. Frequent and regular feeding helps to over come this.

Feeding should be done after proper cleaning of the breasts. Breasts should be washed or wiped with a wet cloth just before and just after feeding.

Feeding should be done in the proper position.The best position is with the mother sitting upright with proper support for her back, holding the baby with its head supported by her arm on the side of the breast to be fed and the baby's chin touching the breast. The mother has to guide the nipple and areola into the baby's mouth. It's better not to lie down during the feed as it could choke the baby. This contact during breast feeding establishes a strong mother-child relationship.

Long hours of not feeding could cause engorgement of breast giving severe pain and tenderness. So to prevent this, periodical feeding or draining of the accumulated milk should be done. In very severe cases the milk solidifies and leads to inflammation of the ducts etc. where minor surgical procedures might be needed. Warm fomentation done to the breasts can solve this easily. Aloe vera gel and turmeric applications on the breast help too. Pulp of roots of bitter gourd crushed and boiled in water, is also beneficial. According to Ayurveda, a mother's milk should be fed to the baby initially. If that is unavailable, then diluted milk from a goat or cow, boiled with special herbs, could be given.

A new mother should refrain from getting angry or sad. She should not fast either. She should be fed with nourishing food like meat soup, medicated wine etc. She should engage in meditation.

Holistic approach

There are a few herbs prescribed to improve lactation. They are:

- Satavari (Asparagus Racemosus) root powder, taken orally with milk.
- Yastimadhu (Glicyrrhiza Glabra) taken with sweetened milk.
- Aswagandha (Withania Somnifera).

Pumpkin, leaves of drumstick, Jeevanti (Leptadenia Reticulate), Pippali (Piper Longum) should also be included. Traditional healers suggest roasted jeera (cumin seeds) in the food. In case lactation needs to be suppressed, jasmine flowers, and cabbage leaves could be placed on the breast.

To regain the shape of the breasts after lactation, a paste made of roots of Mimosa Pudika and Aswagandha should be applied.

Homeopathy

Ricinus Communis and Urtica Urens are good remedies for increasing milk production in females with this problem.

Naturopathy

During lactation, naturopathy advises foods rich in calcium and protein. This includes whole grains, milk and its products, soya and its products, all vegetables and fruits.

Meditation, deep relaxation techniques, and pranayamas too help in de-stressing and ensure proper lactation.

Ayurveda

Cosuming a lot of milk, milk boiled with Aswagandha, black gram, Vidarayadi Lehyam, Panchajeeraka Gudam, and Aswagandhadi Lehyam help. Also one should include drumstick leaves in one's diet.

Uterine Prolapse

Uterine prolapse is the falling or sliding of the womb (uterus) from its normal position into the vaginal area.

Causes

Muscle weakness or relaxation may let the uterus sag or come completely out of the body to a variable degree.

Conditions like multiple pregnancies, weakness of pelvic muscles, obesity, chronic coughs which causes increase in intra-abdominal pressure, excessive weightlifting etc. are responsible for uterine prolapse.

Common symptoms

- ❖ A feeling of fullness or pressure in the pelvis (it may be described as a feeling of sitting on a small ball).
- ❖ Lower back pain.
- ❖ Feeling that something is coming out of the vagina.
- ❖ Painful sexual intercourse.
- ❖ Difficulty in urination or bowel movement.
- ❖ Difficulty in walking.

Prevention

- ❖ Kegel exercises: To strengthen the pelvic muscles.

- Diet: To reduce the weight if the prolapse is because of obesity.
- Avoid excessive weightlifting.
- Treat first the factors which cause increased intra-abdominal pressure such as chronic coughs.
- Physical hygiene to prevent infections.

Holistic approach

Homeopathy

The medicines will help in strengthening the pelvic muscles. Homeopathic medicines help to prevent further prolapse and also have a great role in preventing complications such as infection, urinary discomfort, and lower back pain.

Naturopathy

Naturopathic treatments like T-pack, hip bath, douches, and acupuncture help too.

Ayurveda

Ayurvedic treatments like Vasti, herbal hip baths, Kizhis, and Abhyanga strengthen the muscles and prevent prolapse. Treatments also help in fixing the condition and preventing further progress. Ayurvedic internal medications help to strengthen the uterine muscles, ligaments and the pelvic muscles.

Yoga

Yogic postures to strengthen the pelvic floor muscles (described later) should be practiced regularly. These include Baddha Konasana, Upavistakonasana, Bakasana, Vajrasana, and Ashwini mudra help to strengthen the pelvic floor muscles.

How to Shed Weight Gained During Pregnancy

The weight gained during pregnancy varies in each individual. In early weeks of pregnancy, there could be weight loss due to vomiting, nausea, and diminished food intake as well. And hence the weight gain in the 1st trimester could either be nil or just a kilo or two. But later there is a constant gain until the last 2 weeks, when it gets stabilized. The total average weight gain during pregnancy is 10–12 kilos. This gain is partially due to water retention, caused by hormonal changes. This water retained could be up to 6.5 litres.

Generally after deliveries, more than 70 percent of the weight gained during pregnancy is lost. This is the weight of the foetus, the tissues, and the fluid loss. Within the initial week or 10 days, the remaining weight is also lost, which would have been the water retention.

But later as the woman starts to get fed with nourishing food, she starts to gain weight. The metabolism is sluggish, and in combination with inactivity and the happiness of motherhood, one tends to gain a lot of weight. One is also not very keen on the restriction of the quality and quantity of food, as she is lactating and it would affect the child's health. This is also combined with the myth that mothers need double the quantity of food and rich food to meet the demands of the child, whereas in reality, it is a balanced diet which is more important.

Holistic approach

Homeopathy

Kali Carb, Calcarea Carb, Sulphur, Natrum Carb, and Thuja are some medicines that can be used. These should only be taken in consultation with a homeopathic doctor.

Ayurveda

Through treatments and internal medications, the aim is to strengthen the nervous system, to recuperate and rejuvenate the body, to improve the metabolism, and to enable the involution of uterus. These also help to tone the body and prevent excess weight gain. Some times postpartum depression could also contribute to over eating and gain in weight.

The ayurvedic approach helps to fight this depression, especially with treatments like head massages and body oil applications.

Yoga

Meditation and deep breathing help in controlling emotions. They also help to keep the mind relaxed. Yoga asanas should be started after 20 days of delivery. One should start with simple movements and awareness of breathing. After a week's practice, slowly a few advanced postures could be practiced. Asanas mentioned to strengthen the pelvic floor muscles could be practiced. These help to tone the pelvic muscles and cut abdominal flab. They tone the buttock and inner thighs and help to regain the body shape. Internally too, these exercises bring about changes. They help in improving digestion and remove constipation and flatulence. They help in improving the general metabolism as well.

Some of the asanas which are particular advised (apart from the pelvic strengthening) are Yoga Mudrasana, Gomukhasana, Vakrasana, Trikonasana, Sarvangasana, Pawanmuktasana, Padahastasana, Paschimottanasa etc., apart from Suryanamaskar.

Diet

Diet should be satwik in nature. Vegetarian food, freshly cooked with minimum spices, is advised. Water intake should be adequate to flush out the toxins from the system.

As one stops breastfeeding, a conscious effort should be made to reduce the quantity of food intake to half or even less, as otherwise that would mean extra calories, contributing to the weight gain.

Kapha enhancing foods such as dairy products, calcium rich foods, carbohydrates, and proteins should be included. The food should comprise of all 6 tastes namely sweet, sour, bitter, pungent, salty, and astringent. Easily digestible food should be taken so as not to cause indigestion.

Lots of fresh fruits, vegetables, fruit juices, and thin soups should be included.

DR MATHAI'S TIPS

- Brisk walking is encouraged from around 5–6 weeks after delivery.
- However, going to a gym and other strenuous exercises should be started only after 3 months.

Gestational Diabetes

Gestational diabetes is a temporary form of diabetes (high blood sugar) that can develop during pregnancy as a result of hormonal imbalances. Ordinarily, the insulin that pancreas produce allows the body to convert blood sugar into energy but pregnancy hormones can interfere with this process, making the body resistant to insulin and causing your blood sugar levels to rise. The blood sugar levels return to normal after the baby is delivered. Usually there are no symptoms, or if present, are mild and not life threatening to the pregnant woman.

About 4 percent of pregnant women develop gestational diabetes, usually mid-pregnancy, between the 24th and 28th week. It is important to be tested for diabetes around this stage of the pregnancy, or even earlier if they are in a high-risk group. You're more likely to develop gestational diabetes if you're over 25-years-old, have a family history of diabetes, have high blood pressure, are overweight, have too much amniotic fluid, have had an unexplained miscarriage or stillbirth, or were overweight before your pregnancy.

The goals of treatment are to keep blood sugar (glucose) levels within normal limits during the pregnancy, and to make sure that the growing baby is healthy. In general, diet should be moderate in fat and protein and provide controlled levels of carbohydrates through foods that include fruits, vegetables, and complex carbohydrates (such as bread, cereal, pasta and rice). Cut back on foods that contains a lot of sugar, such as soft drinks, fruit juices, and pastries.

Eat three small to moderate sized meals and one or more snacks each day. Do not skip meals and snacks. Keep the amount and types of food (carbohydrates, fats, and proteins) the same from day to day.

If managing diet does not control blood sugar (glucose) levels, one may be prescribed diabetes medicine or insulin therapy while monitoring sugar levels. Most women who develop gestational diabetes will not need diabetes medicines or insulin, but some do.

Holistic approach

An integrated approach that combines the benefits of herbal and homeopathic medicines, naturopathic therapies, yoga therapy is very useful in such conditions. Treatments for gestational diabetes focus on keeping your blood sugar levels in check through proper diet and exercise. Walking and light exercises, while always beneficial in a pregnancy, are even more important in gestational diabetes.

Acupuncture can not only lower blood sugar but also control excessive hunger and thirst, reduce the frequency of urination, improve circulation, and restore proper flow of energy in the body. Herbal remedies help to maintain blood sugar levels, as well as treating the symptoms.

Homeopathy

Gestational diabetes mostly happens in elderly people. Medicines like Phosphorus, Natrum Muriaticumm, and Cal Carb will help in controlling blood sugar. Syzygium Jumbolanum Q, Cephalandra Q, and Gymnema Q can help to control the blood sugar and can be taken along with any allopathic medicine the patient might be taking.

Naturopathy

Reduce direct sugar in the diet and include fenugreek powder, bittergourd etc.

Ayurveda

Nishakadakadi Kashayam could be taken to control the sugar. Drinking water boiled with kadira and dry ginger also helps.

Vomiting During Pregnancy

Vomiting is one of the foremost symptoms of pregnancy. All women experience nausea and vomiting at least few times during their pregnancies. This is caused due to changes in the hormones and the changes in the system due to the growth of the foetus.

Vomiting usually starts with the onset of pregnancy and generally lasts for the 1st trimester. In a few cases, it extends throughout the pregnancy upto the time of labour.

Generally vomiting is experienced immediately on waking up and also a few times during the day. Strong smells and odours, even from food, spices, and sight of certain foods can cause nausea and vomiting.

Vomiting can sometimes create some complications. Uncontrolled vomiting, leading to an inability to hold any food or drink, can cause a lot of exhaustion and malnourishment. This condition is medically called Hyperemis Gravidarum. In very rare cases, this needs proper medical attention.

In some cases, continuous vomiting could indicate grave disease like pre-eclampsia where it is accompanied by high blood pressure, edema, seizures, and hyperproteinemia. This could be a cause for miscarriage and medical termination of pregnancy.

Prevention

- Try to eat some dry carbohydrates like plain crackers or rusks immediately on waking up, even before brushing.
- Drink water with a dash of lime to prevent nausea.
- Eat small quantities of food at regular intervals.
- Eat bland food with very little spices.
- Avoid strong smelling food.

Holistic approach

Homeopathy

Ipecac 30, Symphoricarpus Racemosa 30 or 200 could be taken as and when needed.

Naturopathy

Naturopathic cold packs and compresses relieve acidity and indigestion. Naturopathy advices ice sipping, sipping cold plain milk etc. to prevent vomiting.

Ayurveda

Internal medications like Madiphalarasayanam, water boiled with puffed corn etc. help. Make sure to drink enough water.

INFERTILITY

Conception, pregnancy, and childbirth involve all aspects of physiology, but the involvement of the brain, mind, and the endocrine system are especially important.

Infertility is a condition where a woman is unable to conceive inspite of a normal sexual life.

Causes

The reasons could be many, primarily due to a defect in either the female or male reproductive systems.

Other reasons could be structural deformities, altered pH of the mucosal lining, hormonal disorders like hypothyroidism, polycystic ovarian disease, abnormal sex hormones, estrogen surge, or genetic abnormalities in the female. In the male, the reasons could be reduced sperm count, reduced sperm motility, diminished quality of sperm, and hormonal disorders. Diseases like varicocele too contribute to infertility.

Increased levels of stress contribute a lot to infertility as well. Stress causes the endocrine system to get deranged, leading to impaired secretion of the sex hormones, mainly estrogen and progesterone in women and testosterone in men.

Thoughts too influence fertility. If a woman is doubtful of her ability to be a good mother, her fertility could be diminished, same way as a man who is doubtful or apprehensive of having a child will fail to contribute.

Symptoms

When a woman is in stress, the uterus and the fallopian tubes could get into a spasm, impairing the proper passage and implantation of the egg.

The inability to conceive can cause a lot of disappointment and stress in a female. This stress further contributes to infertility and thus she falls into a vicious cycle.

Women experience loss of self-esteem and guilt and anxiety over disappointing their partner.

Men feel guilty too resulting in relationship problems and reduced sexual activity. All this affects the quality, structure and quantity of the sperm and in addition, problems like impotency and difficulty in ejaculation are experienced. Sexual enjoyment gets affected as the focus is on making a baby, instead of making love. Insomnia and disturbed sleep sets in, influencing the daily rhythm which again, in turn affects the hormone secretion.

Prevention

If a healthy woman and man in the fertile age group with healthy sperm and ovum mate, and if the channels are clear, their mind happy and clear, then they will give birth to a healthy baby.

Holistic approach

Naturopathy

Naturopathic treatments like T-packs, hip baths etc. help to tone the uterine muscles and the birth canal.

Ayurveda

Those with vitiated Vata, Pitta, or Kapha should be treated with appropriate medications and panchakarma treatments.

In stress-related conditions, treatments like Sirodhara, Thalam, and Abhyanga are helpful to relieve stress and strengthen the nervous system.

Herbal hip baths, uttara vasti, and pichu are given to strengthen the female reproductive system. Snehapanam with appropriate medications is done too.

Nasya and Vasti help to detoxify and improve metabolism and immunity.

Any structural or hormonal abnormalities could be treated through proper treatments and internal medications.

Herbs like Abutilon Indica, Aloe Vera, Hibiscus Rosacinensis, Racinus Communis, Soalnum Igrum, Trigonell Fenumgracum, Serraca Asoka, and Mimosa Pudica are used internally.

According to ayurveda, the man should then adhere to a diet consisting mainly of ghee and milk prepared with sweet herbs and the woman to one with oil and black gram. This enhances the quality of sperm and ovum.

Diet

The food we take judges the quality of our tissues, body secretion etc. Eating junk and unhealthy food give unhealthy secretions. So the food should be wholesome and nutritious. It should include all the nutrients required by the body in right proportions. In addition, folic acid and calcium play a greate role. Include a lot of green leafy vegetables for folic acid and calcium. Ragi, milk products, soya, chicken, fish with small bones, and egg could be taken for calcium as well.

DR MATHAI'S TIPS

Regular exercises such as yoga, walking, and swimming are helpful in improving the circulation, to relieve spasm of the muscles and to de-stress.

DIFFERENCE BETWEEN ALLOPATHIC AND HOLISTIC SYSTEMS OF MEDICINE

ALLOPATHIC	HOLISTIC
Focuses on Measurements SYMPTOMS	Focuses on Experience CAUSES and PATTERNS
Disease as Entity PAIN AVOIDING	Disease as Process PAIN READING
General Classified Diagnosis	Specific Individual Needs
Technical Tools	Integrated Therapies
Remedial/Combative/Reactive	Preventive/Corrective /Pro-Active
Crisis Oriented: Occasional Intervention	Lifestyle Oriented: Sustained Maintenance
Radical. Defensive.	Natural. Ecological.
Medicine As Counter-Agent	Medicine As Co-Agent
Side Effects. Chemicals, Surgery, Radiation, Replacement	Low-Risk. Conservative. Organic. Purification, Manipulation, Correction
Emphasis: 'CURE'	Emphasis: 'HEALING'
Speed, Comfort, Convenience	Restoration. Regeneration. Transformation
Practitioner as Authority PACIFYING	Practitioner as Educator ACTIVATING
Patient as Passive Recipient	Patient as Source of Healing
Mechanical/Analytical/ Bio-Physical	Systemic/Multi-Dimensional /Body-Mind-Spirit
Best For: Infectious Diseases, Trauma, Structural Damage, Organ Failure, Emergency, Surgical conditions	Best For: Degenerative, Chronic Stress and Lifestyle Disorders, Systemic Imbalances, Boosting immunity

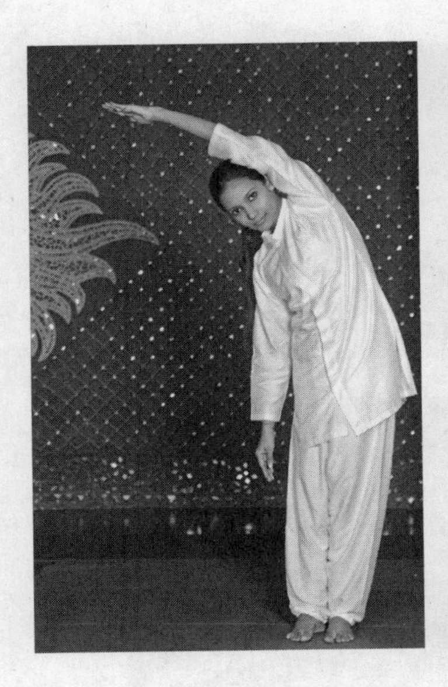

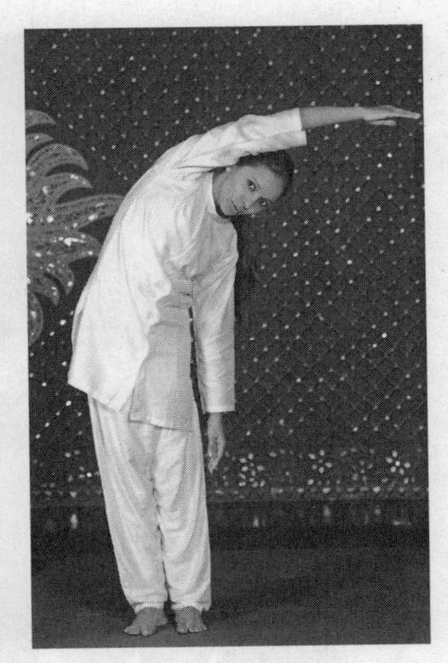

Parswa Chakrasana (lateral arc pose)

- Stand with legs together. Inhale and raise the right arm up.
- Gently push it upwards and exhale and tilt the spine to the left.
- Breathe normally. Feel the stretch in the entire right side of the body and compression in the left hip. Hold for some time.
- With an inhalation, straighten the spine, push up the right arm, exhale, and bring the arm down.
- Feel the mild tingling at the finger tips due to the improved circulation.
- Relax and repeat from the other side.

Benefits

This posture improves the tone of the spine

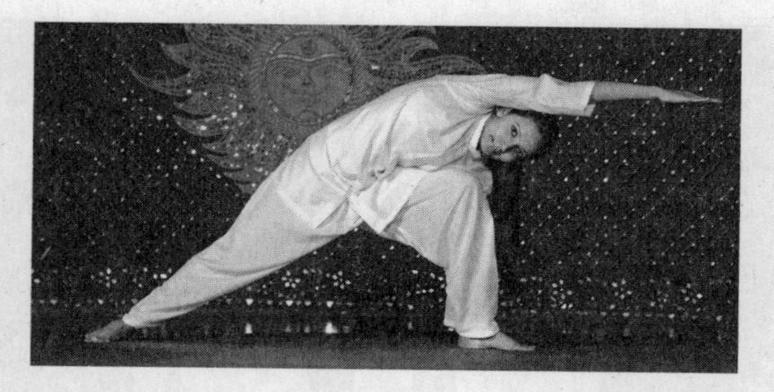

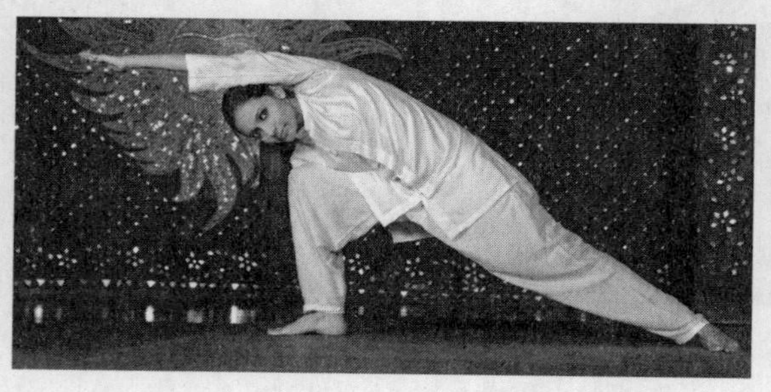

Parswakonasana

- Stand with your legs apart.
- Turn the right foot, toes pointing to the right.
- Bend the right knee at a right angle.
- Bend to the side, to place the right hand by the side of right foot, with an inhalation.
- Let the left arm be lifted, so that the left upper arm touches the left ear with an exhalation.
- Feel the stretch in the inner aspect of the thighs and the pelvic muscles.
- With an inhalation, release the left arm.
- Exhale and straighten the spine and the right leg, release the right hand.
- Relax with the legs apart and practice it on the other side.

Benefits

This asana strengthens the hips, thighs, and tones the abdominal muscles

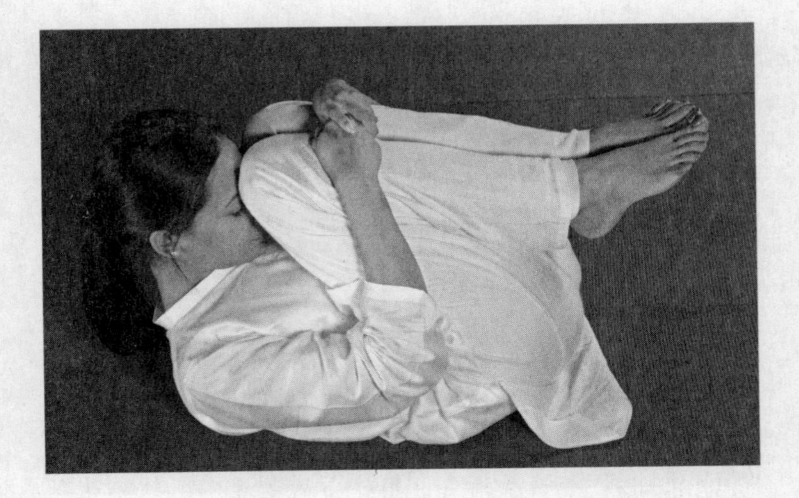

Pawanmuktasana (embryo pose)

- Lay on the back with knees bent and soles of the feet touching the ground.
- With an inhalation, lift the feet up and encircle the knees with the hands.
- Exhale and lift the spine up and try to bring the knees closer to the chest.
- Also try to touch the chin to the knees.
- Hold with normal breathing.
- Feel the relaxation in the lower back.
- Feel the compression and tightening in the abdomen.
- With an inhalation slowly place the head on the ground.
- Exhale and release the legs.

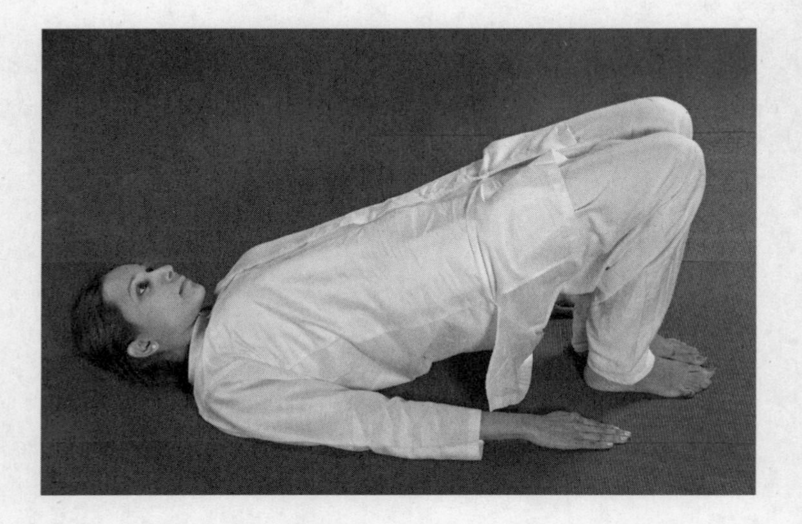

Setubandhasana (bridge pose)

- Lay on the back, bend the legs at the knee, placing the feet on the ground.
- With an inhalation, raise the hips up. Simultaneously, the lumbar region and the thighs will also be raised.
- Hold with normal breathing.
- If needed you could support the hips with the hands.
- Now slowly move the feet forward to give the body, the shape of a perfect bridge.
- With exhalation, slowly place the hips on the ground, straighten the knees and relax.

Benefits

This posture relieves back pain, relaxes the spine and the muscles by the side of the spine

CHAPTER SEVEN

Menopause

MENOPAUSE IS THE CULMINATION OF ONE'S FERTILE life, when ovulation ceases and so does menstruation. This generally occurs between 45–50 years of age. However it varies depending upon factors such as heredity, stress, medications, and illnesses.

Menopause is a cessation of the ovarian activity. As a result, functions of many other glands change leading to the various symptoms associated with menopause.

Common symptoms

As menopause sets in, the female reproductive system gets shrunken and atrophied as a result of inactivity and hormonal changes. The external genitalia too shows some changes.

As a result of the laxed muscles and ligaments, there are more chances for the uterus to prolapse. The breasts get atrophied and pendulous. The skin wrinkles. Arthritic changes develop in the joints and there could be a rise in blood pressure, palpitations, and/or tachycardia.

Hot flushes are felt more towards evenings with profuse sweating, lasting for about 10–15 minutes. Sleep could get disturbed too. Digestive disturbances like flatulence, constipation etc. are also common.

Some people complain of pins and needles in the extremities. Sexual feelings generally get increased with menopause. Headaches, irritability, depression, and melancholia are common.

The absence of menstruation along with presenting symptoms can sometimes mimic pregnancy and is called pseudocyecis.

Types

There are three ways by which menstruation ceases.

- ❖ It could be a sudden stop of bleeding, never to return.
- ❖ The cycles could be regular, but the bleeding reduces gradually. Sometimes the gap between periods could get longer and ultimately stop. These is considered quite normal.
- ❖ But if any heavy bleeding occurs or the periods get too frequent, other pathological conditions, especially cancer, should be ruled out.

All the above said symptoms arise only because of the change in hormones. So hormone replacement is recommended usually. As a result of the hormonal changes, dryness of vagina, frequent urinary tract infections etc. set in. The reduced level of estrogen can interfere with the calcium metabolism too, making the bones brittle.

Prevention

- ❖ Weight-bearing exercises, walking, and yogic stretches help the strengthening of bones and joints.
- ❖ Pranayama and meditation help calm the mind and control moods.
- ❖ Eating a wholesome diet with a good amount of calcium can keep the bones strong. This includes skimmed milk

products, spinach and all green leaves, ragi, oats, soya and its products etc.

❖ Food containing phyto-estrogens like soya and its products, fennel, alfalfa, and flaxseeds should be consumed

Holistic approach

Homeopathy

Lachesis, Calcarea Carb, Sulphur, Graphytis, Calcarea Phos, Sepia, Pulsatilla, and Ignatia can be given as constitutional homeopathic medicines.

Lachesis 200, Sulphur 1m, and Belladona 200 are good medicines for hot flashes. Calcarea phosphoricum 6x can be taken to maintain the calcium level.

Naturopathy

General body massages, immersion baths, and hip baths help improve the body condition. Regular body massage with aromatic oils and medicated oils help pass through the phase in a easier way.

Ayurveda

Treatments like Sirodhara, Abhyanga etc. help to set right the hormonal imbalance and to calm the mind to enable sleep better.

Giloy Satwa is helpful to control hot flushes. Chandanasavam can also be taken.

Yoga

Yogic postures and pranayamas such as Brahmari, Ujjayi, and Nadi Shodhana help to keep the mind relaxed and calm. Meditation helps in keeping the mind and emotions under control.

How to Maintain Youthfulness

Youthfulness is a state of mind. This mind state usually affects our physiology and appearance as well. Age is just a number and our body is actually much younger than we think.

Having said this, health is an important aspect of feeling young. When one is in a complete state of physical, mental, and emotional harmony, one feels active and young. Health is a state of being that can be achieved by following some easy steps and taking a bit of extra care of oneself.

Food is an important aspect of our daily needs. Good nutrition cannot be substituted by anything else. To get a balanced diet and nutrition, it is important to choose foods from all food groups. Eating a varied diet increases the chances of all nutrient needs being met.

Proteins, carbohydrates, and fats are the macronutrients that the body needs to maintain and regulate body functions. Most people doing average activity in a day should get approximately 50 percent of their daily calories from carbohydrates, 15 percent to 20 percent from proteins, and 30 percent from a fat source. Our body contains about 60–75 percent water. Even though we do not realize it, water is an important component of proper nutrition. It is needed for several key functions like regulation of temperature, transport and absorption of nutrients, and elimination of waste products from the body.

Another important aspect of maintaining youthfulness is regular exercise. This increases vitality, improves metabolism and body functions, and helps in maintaining the ideal weight. It is more helpful to have a fixed time to do exercise on a regular basis. Practices like yoga, breathing exercises etc. work on the mind and body as well help to maintain a balance in life.

Hobbies like active sports, art and theatre, listening to good music and dancing help to maintain youthfulness.

Being in the company of the young and engaging in interesting conversations also help maintain youthfulness of the mind. Keeping abreast with the latest developments in the society, technical advancements, and making an effort to learn and use new gadgets is also a part of youthfulness.

As one ages, their skin tends to get dry. Regular mositurising using milk cream, glycerine, and rose water mixture prevents wrinkle formation. One should also exercise the facial muscles using gentle movements and exercises.

Using herbal oils like coconut oil boiled with aloe vera, curry leaves, black pepper, and henna leaves will prevent hair fall and delay greying.

Holistic approach

The holistic approach deals with the mind, body, and spirit, enhancing the overall health to maintain youthfulness.

Naturopathy

In addition to a good diet and exercise, some natural packs, mud applications, and fruit packs help to tighten the skin.

Yoga

Yogic postures including the Suryanamaskar series can maintain the suppleness of the body, give a great shape, and maintain erect posture.

As the age advances, one has a tendency to slouch. This in fact would make one appear much older than one actually is. Hence maintaining correct posture is also very critical. Panchakarma after 40s is the best way to keep youthfulness.

Reduced Sexual Urge

Medically it is called lack of libido, or low sex drive. Libido is nothing but the person's sex drive or desire for sexual activity. The desire for sex is an aspect of a person's sexuality, but varies enormously from one person to another. It also varies depending on circumstances at a particular time. The sex drive usually has biological, psychological, and social components. Biologically, levels of hormones such as testosterone are believed to affect sex drive; social factors, such as work and family, also have an impact; as do internal psychological factors like personality and stress. Sex drive may be affected by medical conditions, medications, and lifestyle and relationship issues. A person who has extremely frequent or a suddenly increased sex drive may be experiencing hyper sexuality, but there is no measure of what is a healthy level for sex.

Causes

The root causes usually are psychological stress, depression, fear of getting pregnant, performance anxiety, and frequently boredom—rather than hormonal or physical. There is no 'normal' level of desire for sex (libido) in men or women, although in both sexes it is the 'male' hormone testosterone which sustains it. Testosterone levels can be depressed by poor liver or kidney function, pituitary problems, fatigue, pain, illness, depression, and stress, and also by tranquillizers, opiates, drugs used to treat high blood pressure, appetite suppressants, and alcohol.

The lack of sexual desire could start at the onset of married life or in the later years. One simple reason could be just a dislike towards partner, or the sexual act itself, or body odour, or thoughts of previous acts. Very rarely is it due to hormones. Sometimes it can also be due to deeply rooted false beliefs in the mind about sex.

Stress has a very major role to play. Though good sex is enjoyable and believed to be a great stressbuster, stress could diminish the urge in most cases.

Some women develop low libido after pregnancy and childbirth. The reasons could be either hormonal, fear of pregnancy, or simply reduced levels of energy with the extra care showered on the newborn. Over a period of time, this could turn into a fear of children catching them in the act or lack of privacy.

Counselling and eliciting the exact reason through a detailed evaluation is the key. Based on the results, further counselling, medications, and advices regarding physical comfort can be given.

Holistic approach

Homeopathy

Treatment of underlying conditions mentioned above is the first step to restoring libido. Where cause is mainly psychological, sex therapy can be very helpful. Homeopathic approach is constitutional.

Naturopathy

Treatments like aroma oil massages, aroma therapy etc. help other than dietary and yogic intervention.

Ayurveda

Ayurvedic treatments like Sirodhara, Abhyanga, and internal medications like Vidaryadi Kashayam, herbs like Kapikachu, Narasimha Rasayanam, and Manasamitravatakam help too.

Increased Abdominal Fat

As women go through their middle years, their proportion of fat to body weight tends to increase more than it does in men. This happens more at menopause when extra fat tends to get deposited around the midsection. Even women who don't actually gain weight may still gain inches at the waist.

Fat accumulated in the lower body i.e. hip is mostly subcutaneous and fat in the abdominal area is largely visceral. Where fat can be deposited in a woman's body is influenced by several factors including hereditary and hormones. At menopause, estrogen production decreases and the ratio of androgen to estrogen increases and this shift has been linked to increased abdominal fat after menopause.

Visceral fat yields easily to exercise and diet. Subcutaneous fat located at the waist is often difficult to budge. Weight loss through diet and exercise triggers many changes that have positive health effects.

Fat cells or adipose tissue was initially considered to be just storage of fat which could be used for energy when needed. Research now suggests that fat cells, especially the abdominal fat cells, are biologically active. Actually fat cells are considered to be endocrine organs or glands which produce hormones and other substances that can profoundly affect our health. One such hormone is leptin which is normally released after a meal and dampens appetite. Fat cells also produce the hormone adiponectin which is thought to influence the response of cells to insulin. Although the individual role of hormones is not very clear, it is clear at least that excess body fat, especially abdominal fat, disrupts the normal balance and functioning of these hormones.

Increased abdominal fat is seen to impair the function of the liver as well, making it sluggish. It makes the total cholesterol levels go high and tends to raise the bad cholesterol and lower good cholesterol. It also impairs insulin production and utilization. As a result, diabetes mellitus, hypertension or high blood pressure, atherosclerosis, and stroke could occur. Mentally too one feels sluggish and inactive.

Increased abdominal fat can cause back pains due to the pressure on the lumbar spine. It could also lead to pain in the legs as it gets difficult to bear weight. In people with weak veins, varicosity could set in.

Prevention

- To bring weight under control in general and reducing abdominal fat in particular, one must do regular moderate physical activity of at least 30 minutes to 60 minutes a day.
- Strength training exercises also help fighting abdominal fat.
- Spot exercising, such as doing sit-ups, can tighten abdominal muscles but it won't reduce visceral fat.
- Specific yogic postures like Pawan Muktasana, Ardha Matsyendrasana, Salabhasana, Naukasana, Dhanurasana, and Merudandasana help to reduce abdominal fat.
- It is also important to strengthen the core muscles, through postures such as Bhujangasana, Salabhasana, Sarpasana, and Parswa Konasana.
- Diet is also important. One should eat foods less in fat and more in fibre. Avoid junk food and deep fried foods completely.
- Avoid sitting immediately after meals. Try to walk slowly for 10–15 minutes after meals.
- Do not sleep immediately after a meal.
- Restrict the intake of carbohydrates and fat at dinner. Take a light meal, both in quantity and quality.

Holistic approach

Homeopathy

Homeopathic medicines help in improving the metabolism and also in reducing adamant weight. Phytolacca Berry is one such medicine. Medicines like Calc Carb, Lycopodium, Nat Carb, and Medorrhinum help in reducing weight too. These medicines are given by doctors after a complete homeopathic health evaluation.

Naturopathy

Naturopathic treatments like hip baths, abdomen compresses, and liver packs help too, in addition to diet and yoga practices.

Ayurveda

Ayurvedic treatments like Udvarthanam, Choorna Swedam, Patrapotala Swedam, and Vasti help improve the body metabolism and reduce abdominal fat. Internal medications are given to improve the metabolism and help in mobilization of fat.

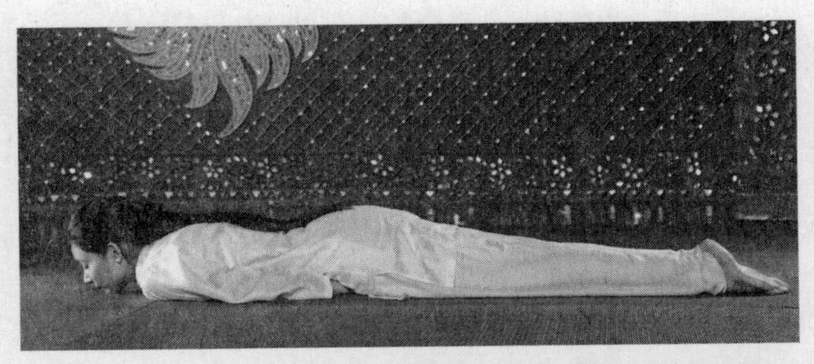

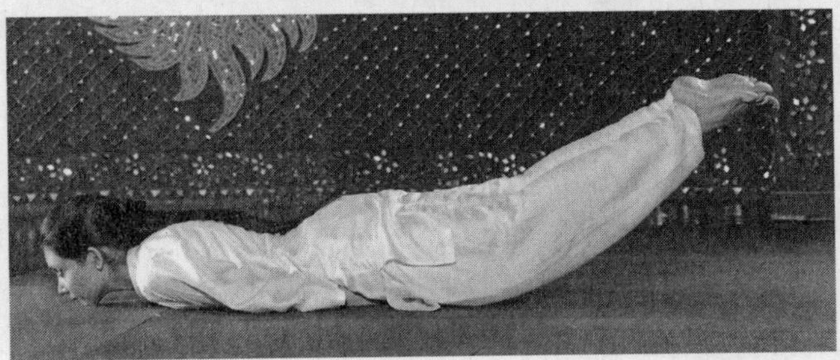

Salabhasana (locust pose)

- Lie on the abdomen with legs together.
- Make fists with the hands and place them beneath the respective thighs, palmar aspect touching the thighs.
- With an inhalation raise the legs up from the thighs, without bending the knees.
- Let the chin be touching the ground.
- You could push the thighs up with the fists if needed.
- Feel the stretch from the lower back to the toes.
- Feel the compression in the abdomen.
- Maintain the pose with normal breathing.
- With exhalation, slowly bring the legs back to the ground.
- Keep the legs apart, release the hands and cross them in front of the body to form a cushion for the face.
- Let the whole body relax.

Benefits

This posture relieves the stiffness of the back, strengthens the sciatic nerves, and reduces abdominal fat

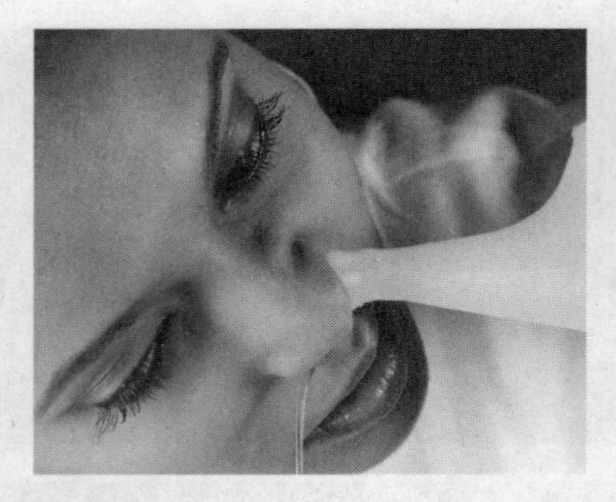

Shatkriyas

Shat means six and karma or kriya means action. These are the 6 purificatory techniques advocated in Hatha yoga

The six techniques are likewise:

Neti, Dhauti, Nauli, Basti, Kapalabhati, and Trataka.

1. Neti is the process of cleansing the nasal passages and the frontal sinuses. The two types of Neti are the Jalaneti (done with water) and Sutraneti (using fine rubber catheters), in the modern days.
2. Dhauti are a series of methods or techniques used to cleanse the internal organs, mainly the alimentary canal. The techniques are sankha prakshalana and laghu sankha prakshalana, agnisara, kunjal kriya and vatsara dhauti. All these are higher practices and should be done only under an expert's guidance and in recommended conditions.
3. Nauli is a method of internal massage and strengthening of the abdominal organs.
4. Basti is done to clean and tone the large intestine.
5. Kapalabhati is considered both a shatkarma and a pranayamas. This stimulates and cleanses the frontal region of the brain. Since breathing is incorporated in the technique, it's considered a pranayama as well.
6. Trataka is a practice, where intense gazing on a fixed point is done to improve the concentration.

All the above need practice. It should be done only when the yoga teacher finds it right for you to do it. It should be attempted initially, only in the presence of the teacher. These techniques should never be done reading a book or after watching videos.

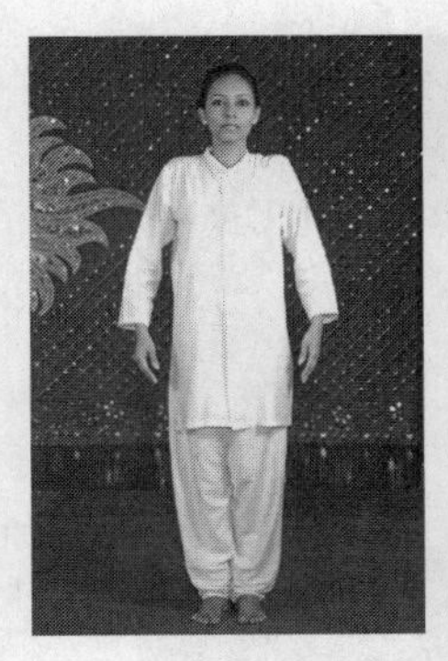
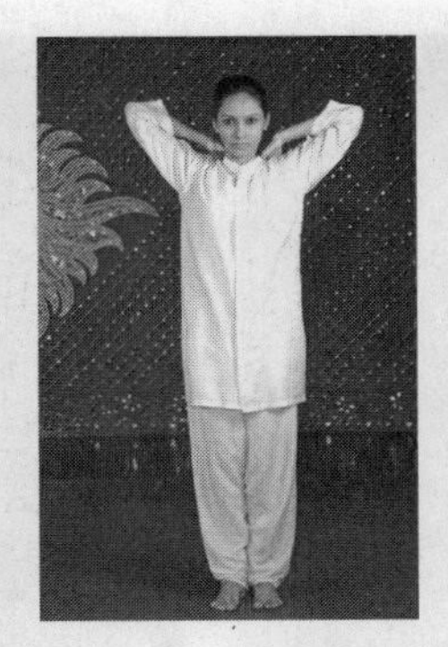
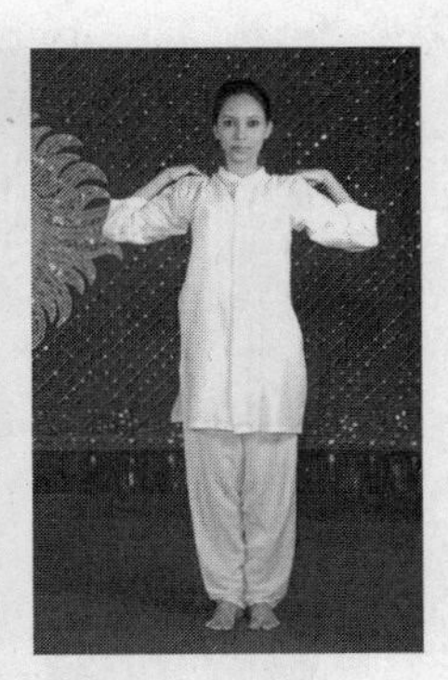
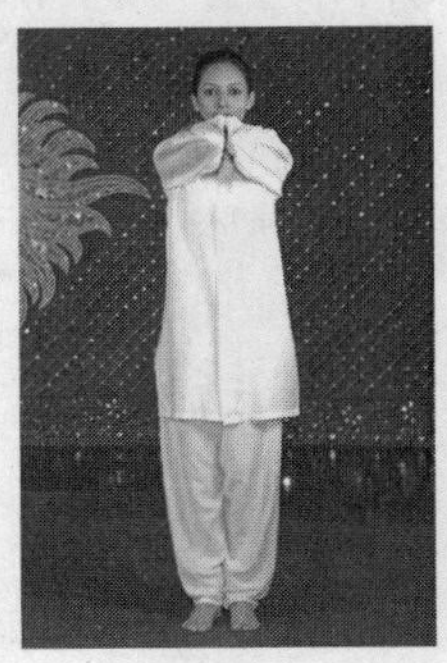
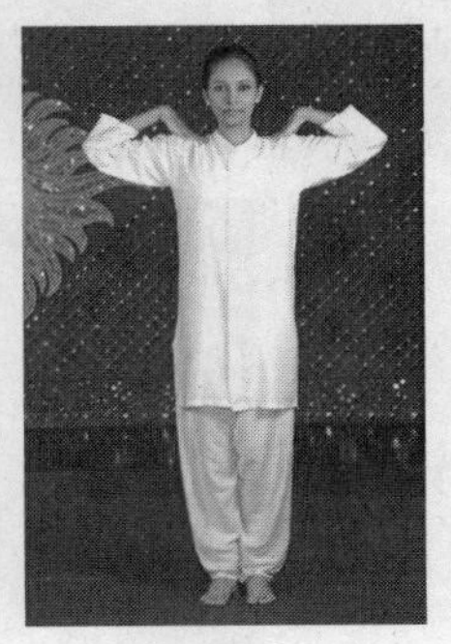

Shoulder Movements

1. Shrugging: When you inhale, raise the shoulders up and as you exhale gently release them. Feel the compression in the muscles around the neck, upper back region and the shoulders. You can also feel the stiffness from the neck and shoulders getting relieved, as you release the shoulders.
2. Bend the elbows, and place the fingers on the respective shoulder. Bring the elbows closer. With inhalation, widen them apart and with exhalation bring them closer. You can feel the stretch and compression in the shoulders as well as the thoracic region.
3. From the above position, take the elbows backwards as you inhale and bring them forward as you exhale to complete a rotation. After 5 rounds, do the movement in the opposite direction.
4. You can feel the effect of the massage on the muscles around the shoulder joint.

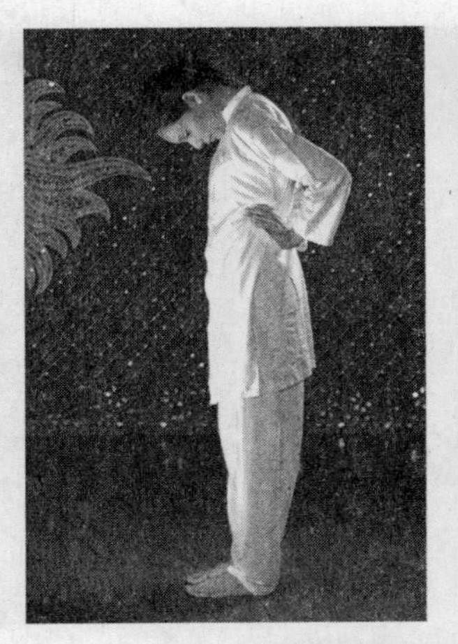

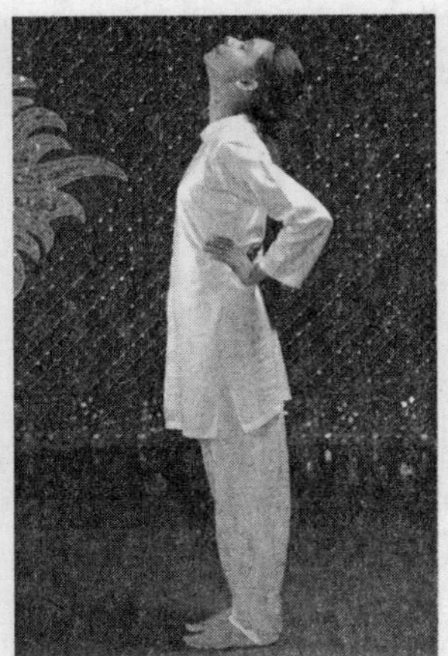

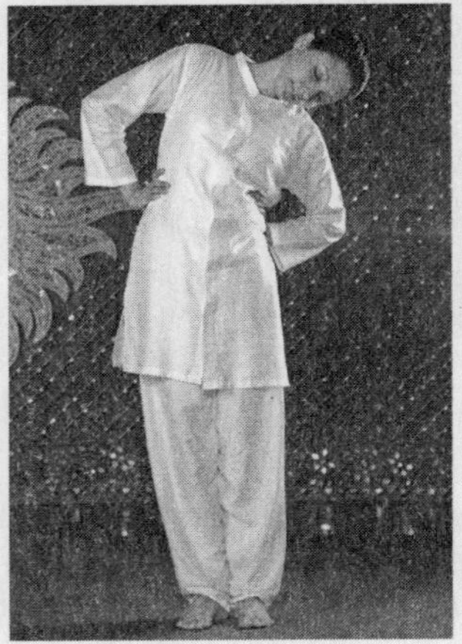

Spinal Movements

1. Backward and forward bending of the spine. Inhale, bend backwards and exhale and bend forward without bending the hips. You feel complete stretch and compression in the spine and the muscles by the side of the spine.
2. Now take a deep inhalation and as you exhale bend to one side, inhale and come up; exhale and tilt to the other side, inhale and come up. You feel the stretch laterally in the spine and the muscles by the side of the spine.

CHAPTER EIGHT

Other General Issues

Skin Pigmentation

THE COLOUR OF THE SKIN DEPENDS UPON A SKIN PIGMENT called melanin. Melanin is produced by special cells called melanocytes. Fair-skinned people produce very little melanin, darker-skinned people produce moderate amounts, and very dark-skinned people produce the most. People with albinism have little or no melanin.

Skin pigmentation is mainly because of uneven production of the melanin by melanocytes.

Types

- Sunburn/skin tan: When exposed to sunlight, melanocytes produce increased amounts of melanin, causing the skin to darken or tan.
- Freckles: Some melanocytes produce more melanin than others in reaction to the sunlight and it causes freckles. A tendency to freckles runs in families. Freckles are tiny hyperpigmented spots on the skin.
- Hypopigmentation: Melanocytes produce very low amount of melanin and it affects a large part of the body. Decreased

melanin usually results from a previous injury to the skin, such as a blisters, ulcers, burns, or skin infections.

- Hyperpigmentation: Melanocytes produce large amount of melanin which causes itching, thickness, and dark patches on the skin. Few examples of hyperpigmentation are stretch marks after pregnancy, lichen planus chronicus, scars after injuries, and Addison's disease. During pregnancy the hormone levels may increase the melanin production.
- Post menopause too due to the changes in the hormones, some tend to get pigmentation on the face, upper back, elbows, and neck.
- This pigmentation could set in during pregnancy, again due to the hormones, but tends to disappear immediately after delivery.
- Liver diseases cause pigmentation as well.
- Skin pigmentations can occur due to allergy to certain cosmetics.

Prevention

Avoid direct sun exposure and make sure the body is fully covered when exposed to the sun.

Holistic approach

The main approach is to detoxify the system through ayurvedic and naturopathy treatments and internal medications. Detoxification ensures proper functioning of the internal organs and strengthens each and every cell in the body. This will set right all the physical causes. Detoxification also works at the mental level and clears emotions, making the person calm, which reflects on the skin.

Proper diet also plays a major role in protecting the skin and preventing damage. Diet high in vitamins and minerals to nourish the skin include wheatgrass juice, carrot juice, ample intake of water and fluids, avoiding fatty and junk food etc.

Homeopathy
According to the theory of homeopathy, skin disorders are the reflections of internal issues and should be treated by giving medicines internally. Homeopathic medicines help in regulating the hormonal imbalance and also in controling the regulation of melanin production. The skin tone and texture then gets balanced with homeopathic medicines. The occurrences for new patches on skin will reduce and then stop completely.

Naturopathy
Herbal packs with mint leaves, turmeric, and various herbal mud packs help the pigmentation.

Ayurvedic
Ayurvedic facials using Navara rice, Manjishta, Lodhra, and internal medications like Manjistadi Kashayam, Sukumaram Kashayam, and Saaribadyasavam are helpful.

Yoga
Exercises help to improve oxygenation to the skin and maintain the texture. Asanas, pranayamas, and meditation are particularly beneficial as they directly influence the skin through a good oxygen supply.

Kitchen cures
There are certain natural home remedies to help pigmentation.

- Washing face with curd after sun exposure will relieve pigmentation.
- Face packs made with chickpea flour, drops of lemon juice, egg white, honey, and turmeric can reduce pigmentation.
- Papaya, potato, and carrot paste on the face helps too.
- Lemon juice with honey applied on the face gives bleaching effect.
- Red sandal powder can take way pigmentation.

- Milk cream with kasturi turmeric applied can also relieve pigmentation.

Haemorrhoids

Haemorrhoids are swollen veins in the anal canal. This common problem can be painful, but it's usually not serious. Too much pressure on the veins in the pelvic and rectal area causes this issue.

Causes

Normally, the tissue inside the anus fills with blood to help control bowel movements. If you strain to move stool, the increased pressure causes the veins in this tissue to swell and stretch. This can cause haemorrhoids. Diarrhoea or constipation also may lead to straining and can increase pressure on the veins in the anal canal.

Pregnant women can get haemorrhoids during the last 6 months of their pregnancy. This is because of the increased pressure on the blood vessels in the pelvic area. Straining to push the baby out during labor can make haemorrhoids worse.

Being overweight can also lead to haemorrhoids.

Common Symptoms

The most common symptoms of both internal and external haemorrhoids include:

- Bleeding during bowel movements. You might see streaks of bright red blood on toilet paper after you strain to have a bowel movement.
- Itching rectal pain. It may be painful to clean the anal area.

Types

Internal haemorrhoids

With internal haemorrhoids, you may see bright red streaks of blood on toilet paper or bright red blood in the toilet bowl after you have a normal bowel movement. You may see blood on the surface of the stool.

Internal haemorrhoids often are small, swollen veins in the wall of the anal canal. But they can be large, sagging veins that bulge out of the anus all the time. They can be painful if they bulge out and are squeezed by the anal muscles. They may be very painful if the blood supply to the haemorrhoids is cut off. If haemorrhoids bulge out, you also may see mucus on the toilet paper or stool.

External haemorrhoids

External haemorrhoids can get irritated and clot under the skin, causing a hard painful lump. This is called a thrombosed, or clotted, haemorrhoids.

Signs and tests

Your doctor can tell if you have haemorrhoids by asking about your past health and doing a physical exam.

You may not need many tests at first, especially if you are younger than 50 and your doctor thinks that your rectal bleeding is caused by haemorrhoids. Your doctor may just examine your rectum with a gloved finger. Or your doctor may use a short, lighted scope to look inside the rectum.

Holistic approach

For most external haemorrhoids, home treatments are all you need. This includes slowly adding fibre to your meals and drinking more water. Healthy habits can help you prevent haemorrhoids or keep them from getting worse. Eat foods that have lots of fibre such as fruits, vegetables, and whole grains. Also, drink plenty of water, and get plenty of exercise. You also may use natural stool softeners like husks, papaya, and leafy vegetables.

Homeopathy
Aesculus can be used for large bluish painful haemorrhoids which are accompanied by back pain. Aloes can be taken for haemorrhoids that look like a bunch of grapes and cause stick like pain in the rectum and lose stools. Acid Nit can be used for bleeding haemorrhoids with burning pains. Ratanhia is a good remedy for haemorrhoids with a lot of pain that lasts for a long duration after the stool. Nux Vom can be used for protruding piles combines with constipation and an ineffectual desire for stool.

Naturopathy
Therapies like hip baths, cold bidet, ice applications, and cold douches help stop the bleeding and regress the mass.

Ayurveda
Depending on whether the piles are bleeding or dry, the treatments will differ. Fomentation with black gram and horse gram is given to reduce the swelling and the inflammation. This is followed by herbal hip baths, which reduce the mass of the pile. Fumigation with herbs such as Vidanga or Devadaru is helpful. Diet to improve digestion and excretion is prescribed. This includes green gram soup, yam with pepper, brown rice, milk and all types of nourishing food. If the piles are bleeding, cold oil massages, jets of cold water, and application of ghee help. Herbal hip baths with Mimosa Pudika, lotus petals, and white sandal is also good. Buttermilk is very good and should be included in meals regularly.

Chiruvilvadi Kashayam, Gandharvahastadi Kashayam,

Hinguvachadi Choornam, Vaiswanarachoornam, Manibhadra Gulam, Kalyanagulam are all prescribed.

Reduced Calcium and Vitamin D

Vitamin D and calcium deficiencies are positively correlated to each other. If there is a reduction in Vitamin D, it causes a reduction in calcium levels too. Vitamin D is important in the maintenance of calcium levels in the body. There are 2 types of Vitamin D: D2 and D3; Vitamin D2 is available in all vitamin supplements and Vitamin D3 is available in natural form.

Calcium is a major component of our bones. When calcium levels drop, parathyroid hormone (PTH) is released and it causes the release of calcium from our bones. Because of this, calcium deficiencies often develop.

Vitamin D is important to enable absorption of calcium intobody and also for the maintenance of calcium and phosphate. Vitamin D regulates calcium absorption and its excretion when the levels are low.

Common symptoms

Bone pains, muscular weakness, recurrent fractures, petechiae, pins and tingling sensation in oral cavity, rickets, osteomalacia, and osteoporosis are the symptoms of calcium and Vitamin-D deficiency.

Generally, after menopause, women tend to be deficient of calcium. This is because of the depleting level of estrogen causing the calcium to be absorbed from the bones.

Most of the times general weakness or tiredness or mild pains or aches in the body is neglected. The deficiency could be diagnosed only through proper blood tests. So it is important for a person to undergo the required tests after 40–45 years.

Prevention

Though it is possible to supplement the required calcium through diet, exercise, and sun exposure, the majority of it needs to be supplemented synthetically.

Natural sources of Vitamin D include fish liver oils (cod liver oil), fatty fish (catfish, salmon, mackerel, sardines, tuna, eels), eggs, and shiitake mushrooms, which are one of a few natural sources of vegan Vitamin D.

Exposing onesself to sunlight, between 7 and 9 am in the mornings and 5–6.30 pm in the evenings, without applying any sunscreen helps to improve Vit-D levels in the body.

Calcium is mainly absorbed through milk and milk products. At the stage of menopause, women need to drink 500 ml of milk to supplement the RDA of calcium. Soya milk, ragi, spinach, drumstick leaves, seeds and nuts, small fish with tiny chewable bones, chicken with tender bones are all good sources of calcium.

Weight-bearing exercises improve bone density and thereby prevent the most dangerous symptom of calcium deficiency namely osteoporosis, where the bones get porous and brittle.

Holistic approach

Homeopathic and ayurvedic internal medications helps set right hormonal imbalance, if any, and improve calcium absorption and supplement necessary calcium.

Since calcium and Vit-D deficiencies do not always occur due to deficient intake, but also because of faulty metabolisms, investigations should be done mainly focusing on diet, hormones and digestion. The treatments should also be planned so as to improve the metabolism and correct the hormones and digestion. Dietary modifications are also done.

Homeopathy

Constitutional medicines can be prescribed only after thorough evaluation of the case.

Naturopathy

Naturopathic treatments like liver packs, gastro hepatic packs, and hip baths help improve metabolism.

Ayurveda

Ayurvedic treatments like Navarakizhi, Nasya, and Vasti too help in improving the bone density and setting right the metabolism.

Internal medications are given to improve the calcium and Vit-D absorption like Bone Tone, Gandha Thailam and Dhantawantaram Kashayam.

Diet

Your diet should include calcium-rich foods such as leafy vegetables, ragi, soya and its products, oats, skim milk products, green gram, and fish with small bones.

For Vit-D, though sun exposure is mainly advised, food such as fortified milk, fish such as mackerel, herring, sardines, egg yolk, flaxseeds are to be included.

Water Retention

Water retention, also known as fluid retention, refers to an excessive build-up of fluids in the circulatory system, body tissues, or cavities of the body. Up to 70 percent of the human body consists of water which exists both inside and outside our body's cells. Blood is mostly made up of water, as are our organs and muscles.

Common symptoms

Water retention is generally noticed due to swelling of the feet and hands, swelling of the fingers making finger rings tight, puffiness of the face, and feeling of heaviness. These are noticed mostly on waking up in the mornings, or after a long travel. Inactivity makes it worse. Generally as the day progresses, the swelling or the retention gets better.

Types

In women closer to menstruation and during pregnancy, water retention is noticed, mainly due to the hormonal changes and circulatory reasons.

Water retention is also noticed in some renal diseases, diseases of the heart including hypertension, certain liver disorders, hormonal disorders involving thyroid, or ADH.

Prevention

Cutting down on salt and increasing water intake is the simplest way to get rid of water retention. Diuretics like barley water, tender coconut water, green tea, juice of the stem of plantain tree etc. could be included. If the cause is the involvement of other systems or organs, then it should be treated appropriately. One home remedy is to raise the feet above the level of head, by placing them on propped up pillows, while you sleep.

Physical activity (exercise) helps the leg veins return blood to the heart (against gravity).

Exercise is also needed to stimulate the lymphatic system to fulfill its function of regulating overflow—bringing fluids back into the bloodstream at rates which may regulate body water levels. Very long periods of physical inactivity, such as a long-haul flight, increase the risk of water retention. During a long-haul flight even minor physical movements, such as standing on tiptoes a few times, rotating the ankles, and wiggling the toes can help reduce fluid retention.

Humans require a certain level of proteins for effective water balance. An individual with severe protein deficiency may find it harder to get the water from the tissue spaces back into the capillaries. The enlarged abdomens of seriously malnourished and/or starving people are mainly caused by a lack of protein in their diet.

Holistic approach

Acupuncture, auriculotherapy, kidney packs, GH packs, wet packs, under water massages, specific dietary regulations, yoga therapy, colonic irrigation, steam baths—all these intend to remove the excess water retention by stimulating the excretory organs. Homeopathic remedies, ayurvedic internal medicines and therapies like Choorna Swedam and Vasti are useful in such conditions.

Homeopathy

Apis is good for generalized edema or swelling of the body. The other medicines are Calcarea Carb, Thuja, Kali Carb, and Graphites. These are to be taken only in consultation with a homeopathic physician.

Naturopathy

Treatments to improve seating and recucing water retention like steam baths, Turkish baths, under water massages, and full wet sheet packs are done. Alternate hot and cold immersions help relieve water retension too. In some cases mud application is beneficial as well.

Dietary changes like including plantain pith juice and ash gourd juice help relieve water retention.

Ayurveda

To correct the electrolyte imbalance, circulation has to be improved through massages like Choorna Swedam, PPS, leg massages with special combination of oils, and herbal paste applications. Herbs like Gokshura, Punarnava, ginger and jaggery, Brihatyadikashayam, Punarnavadi Kashayam, Kokilaksham Kashayam are all helpful.

Dry Eyes

Dry eyes occur when the natural phenomenon of lachrymation or tear secretion gets affected. Tears lubricate the eyes and also help fight allergens and infections.

Causes

Dryness is usually felt as a result of sleeplessness, severe allergy, exposure to extreme cold wind/weather, and after rubbing eyes continuously. Sometimes it also happens due to certain infections.

Certain eye cosmetics could also cause dryness.

Dryness is also caused by using contact lens for long hours. It is seen as a symptom of certain auto-immune disorders.

Prevention

- ❖ Wash your eyes regularly with pure rose water/triphala decoction.
- ❖ Remove eye makeup as soon as you are done with it.
- ❖ Never go to bed with eye makeup on.
- ❖ Use cucumber slices or rose water pads on your eyes while you rest.

Holistic approach

Yogic Kriyas, Pranayama, eye packs, vegetable and fruit packs, yogic eye execises, Trataka, Netra Tarpana, herbal remedies, eye drops, ayurvedic treatments are all useful in improving circulation of the fluid in the eyes.

A diet rich in Vit-A is also helpful to the eyes.

Homeopathy

Pulsatilla can help with dryness of eyes. Belladona can be used when there is redness of the eyes along with dryness.

Naturopathy

Mud packs on the eyes will strengthen the muscles. Yogic technique like Trataka and eye exercises improve lubrication.

Ayurveda

Herbal eyedrops and medications to improve lachrymation are prescribed. Treatments like Netra Tarpanam help too.

Bloatedness

Abdominal bloating is a condition in which the tummy feels full, tight, and distended. Belching, flatulence, and bowel movements relieve the symptom of bloating in most the cases.

The bowel of a normal person contains about 200 ml of gas. About 600 ml of gas is evacuated as flatus every day. The five main gases found in the bowel are nitrogen, oxygen, carbon dioxide, hydrogen, and methane. Of these, nitrogen and oxygen are derived from swallowed air and the remaining gases are formed due to fermentation processes by bacteria in the large intestines. The excess gas in the upper gastrointestinal tract is released by belching. Flatulence is the involuntary release of gas from the lower gastrointestinal tract.

DID YOU KNOW?

On an average, a healthy individual passes flatus 14 times per day. Some even report 25 expulsions.

Bloating is the perception of retained excess gas within the lumen of the gut. Women report bloating more often than men. Although some conditions lead to increased gas production, many individuals with bloating exhibit normal gut gas volumes.

Causes

A majority of the conditions that lead to bloating are not serious and include conditions like aerophagia in which abdominal bloating is caused by subconscious swallowing of air.

Most times, abdominal bloating results from a disorder of the function of the gastrointestinal tract. Abdominal bloating could be due to any of the following causes:

- Subconscious swallowing of air—This is called aerophagia. This usually occurs during rapid eating and drinking, chewing gum, smoking, and wearing loose dentures. This is more pronounced in nervous individuals. Most of the upper intestinal air is accumulated because of aerophagia.
- Irritable bowel syndrome—This is characterized by abdominal pain or discomfort associated with altered bowel habits. In this condition the amount and distribution of gas in the gut will be normal. But due to increased sensitivity, there is increased awareness of gas and bloating. Sometimes certain fibre supplements used to treat irritable bowel syndrome and constipation can cause bloating.
- Constipation—Chronic constipation can cause bloated stomach.

- Small intestinal bacterial overgrowth—This is a condition in which abnormally large amount of bacteria are present in the small intestine. This interferes with digestion and absorption of nutrients and causes symptoms like bloating and diarrhoea.
- Excess gas in the bowels—It could be due to malabsorption of nutrients. This is seen in condition like lactose intolerance. Fatty foods delay emptying of stomach and allows the gas to accumulate, thus causing bloating.
- Abnormal motility of the bowel—Conditions that affect the motility of the bowels can result in prominent gas and bloating.
- Intestinal obstruction—If there is intestinal obstruction, it causes abdominal distention, vomiting, and constipation. It is a more serious condition and immediate medical attention is necessary.

Abdominal bloating sensation need not be always due gas in the bowel. Sometimes the tummy may feel full, tight, and distended in other conditions as well

Holistic approach

The holistic approach is to find out the actual reason for the bloatedness and to correct it through proper exercises and treatments.

This includes treatments from naturopathy, ayurveda, and internal medications from ayurveda and homeopathy.

Dietary aspects and some healthy recipes are incorporated to prevent the symptoms.

Homeopathy

Carbo Veg is a good remedy for bloatedness with lot of belching; the bloatedness is felt mostly in the upper abdomen.

China can be used for generalized bloatedness with weakness. Lycopodium is for bloatedness of lower abdomen.

Naturopathy

Naturopathic approach by diet regulation and fasting, mono-diet fasting, naturopathic treatments like hip baths, castor oil packs, enemas, colonic irrigation, GH packs, Kidney packs done alternatively, wet pack packs for abdomen, yogic techniques like Vaman Dhouti will be beneficial to release the accumulation of gases.

Ayurveda

Ayurvedic treatments like Vasti and internal medications too help overcome bloatedness.

Diet

Dietary changes include some juices like ash gourd juice, ginger water etc. Also going on low starch and protein diets helps eliminate gas.

Eliminating foods such as Bengal gram, potato, tapioca, colocasia, egg, cabbage, and eggplant are seen to be helpful.

Reduced Appetite

A decreased desire to eat is a symptom that is common to numerous medical and psychological conditions. Almost any illness can lead to a decrease in appetite. When severe, decreased appetite can lead to unwanted weight loss and malnutrition. Medically, a decrease in appetite is referred to as anorexia.

The reduced appetite is seen as a symptom due to impaired digestion, or it could merely be due to stress or depression. Very rarely is it due to some serious underlying causes like cancer. It could also be a result of undergoing certain treatments like chemotherapy, radiation, high antibiotic intake or as an after effect of some kinds of fever.

In old age, reduced appetite is a common symptom. Leading a sedentary life could cause reduced appetite. The metabolism gets sluggish as one ages. Bloatedness and other digestive symptoms could also diminish the appetite. Enhancing the liver function through liver detoxification can improve the appetite.

Causes

A decreased appetite is almost always seen among elderly adults, and no cause can be found. However, sadness, depression, grief, or anxiety are common causes of weight loss.

Causes of decreased appetite include:

- After-effects of an illness like a fever, cold etc.
- Stress.
- Some digestive disturbances including constipation.
- Use of certain medications, including antibiotics, chemotherapy drugs, codeine, and morphine.

Cancer may also cause decreased appetite, apart from the various other conditions related to kidneys, liver, heart, and lungs.

Holistic approach

Homeopathy

Alfalfa mother tincture, Tuberculinum, Sulphur, Silicea, Cina can be given to regularize the appetite. Alfalfa tonic helps in improving the appetite in adults and in children. There are other constitutional homeopathic medicines that help in improving appetite and metabolism as well. These need to be taken in consultation with a homeopathic doctor.

Naturopathy

Liver packs, abdomen packs, mud packs, gastro hepatic pack, hip baths, massages, and enemas help to enhance the liver function. Various fasting like water fast, juice fast, mono-diet fast, cleansing diet, and therapies like liver packs, mud packs, mud applications, wet packs for abdomen, Vamana Dhouti, colonic irrigation, enema, specific yogic asanas related to abdomen, and dynamic exercises will surely help.

Ayurveda

Medicines containing musta, shunti (dry ginger), piper longum (pippali), Rasna, piper nigrum (pepper) are all used to improve appetite. This could be as a result of a disease or accumulated toxins (ama). Internal medications to digest and eliminate ama from the system and there by to improve digestion and metabolism are prescribed.

Vaiswanarachoornam, Hinguvachadi Choornam, Shaddharanam Gulika will be helpful in severe toxicity. Otherwise fasting will help.

Diet

Cleansing juices like lemon juice with honey, wheatgrass juice, green juice prepared with celery, spinach, curry leaves, mint leaves help in liver detoxification. A decoction made of dry ginger, pepper, lemon juice in hot water can improve the appetite as well.

Taking a short walk and doing regular yogic exercises can strengthen the digestive system.

TASTELESSNESS

Tastelessness generally occurs after long-standing illnesses, prolonged use of medications including antibiotics, digestive disorders etc. apart from severe stress, and certain diseases affecting the taste sensation on the tongue.

Tastelessness leads to diminished eating, which in turn causes weight loss, and malnutrition.

Holistic approach

The aim is to improve the taste sensation. For this, stimulus is given through various tastes. One should consume food containing all 6 tastes namely sweet, salt, sour, spicy, bitter, and astringent.

Digestion should be improved through various treatments and herbal medications.

Pepper, ginger, cumin, and garlic should be included in the diet to stimulate the taste cells and improve digestion.

A complete detoxification with colon hydrotherapy, followed by a liquid fast, will ensure the return and sharpening of senses including taste.

Specific ayurvedic and homeopathic medications also help to improve the taste sensation and relieve tastelessness.

Homeopathy

Natrum Mur, Pulsatilla, Phosphorus, and Silicea are some of the constitutional homeopathic medicines that are used for tastelessness. The treatment for tastelessness goes with complete homeopathic evaluation and understanding the root cause.

Naturopathy

Ginger juice with honey is given to regain the taste sensation. If a woman is able to fast, she is put on fasting with appropriate juices for a few days, depending on her condition.

Ayurveda

Madiphala Rasayanam helps in regaining taste.

Hypothyroidism

Hypothyroidism is a condition in which the thyroid gland does not make enough thyroid hormones. The thyroid gland is located in the front of the neck just below the voice box (larynx). It releases hormones that control the metabolism.

Causes

The most common cause of hypothyroidism is the inflammation of the thyroid gland which damages the gland's cells. Iodine deficiency is the most common cause of hypothyroidism worldwide.

In iodine-replete individuals, hypothyroidism is frequently caused by Hashimoto's thyroiditis, or otherwise as a result of either an absent thyroid gland or a deficiency in stimulating hormones from the hypothalamus or pituitary.

Stress is known to be a significant contributor to thyroid dysfunction. This can be environmental stress as well as the lesser-considered homeostatic stress such as fluctuating blood sugar levels and immune problems.

Hypothyroidism can result from postpartum (following childbirth) thyroiditis, a condition that affects about 5 percent of all women within a year of giving birth. The first phase is typically hyperthyroidism; the thyroid then either returns to normal, or a woman develops hypothyroidism. Of those, women who experience hypothyroidism associated with postpartum thyroiditis, one in 5 will develop permanent hypothyroidism requiring lifelong treatment.

Congenital hypothyroidism is very rare, accounting for approximately 0.2 percent and can have several causes such as thyroid aplasia or defects in the hormone metabolism.

Common symptoms

Early symptoms:

- Being more sensitive to cold.
- Constipation.
- Depression.
- Fatigue, low energy, slowed activity.
- Heavier menstrual periods.
- Joint or muscle pains.
- Paleness or dry skin.
- Thin, brittle hair or fingernails.
- Weakness.
- Weight gain.

Late symptoms, if left untreated in early stage:

- Decreased taste and smell.
- Hoarseness.
- Puffy face, hands, and feet.
- Slow speech.
- Thickening of the skin.
- Thinning of eyebrows.

Signs and tests

A chest X-ray may show an enlarged heart. Specific blood tests to determine the thyroid hormones and the level of electrolytes in the blood can be done.

Prevention

- Due to slowed down metabolism in hypothyroid patients, it is difficult to lose weight compared to other patients. It is advised that regular exercise and walking will help in maintaining the weight.
- Food like soya and its products, cabbage, cauliflower,

broccoli, and Brussels sprouts are to be restricted as they tend to interfere with thyroid secretion.

- One should try and eat small quantities at regular intervals.

Holistic approach

Homeopathy

Patients in the initial staged of diagnosis can start homeopathy medicines which will help in regularizing the thyroid levels with homeopathic thyroid supplements and also constitutional medicines to stimulate the thyroid gland. This will help in releasing the thyroid hormone.

Chronic patients of hypothyroid who have been on synthetic thyroxine have to continue the dosage as per their physicians' advice. Homeopathic constitutional medicines will be given followed by tapering of the dosage of hypothyroid medicines. This will be managed by an endocrinologist, depending on the readings of the thyroid levels.

In many cases, the patient needs to continue the medicines prescribed by her endocrinologist. Homeopathic constitutional medicines will be only given to stop further complications and maintain the right levels of thyroid so that she will not need larger doses of thyroid supplements. New cases can be cured with homeopathic medicines.

Naturopathy

- Throat packs and compresses are advisable to stimulate under acting thyroid glands.
- General treatments to improve the metabolism like full mud baths, immersion baths, and massages are given.
- Dietary advice is made to deal with the symptoms related to the digestive system, for weight loss etc.

Ayurveda

To stimulate the thyroid glands and to improve the metabolism, treatments like Sirodhara, Choorna Swedam, Nasya, Vasti and external application of herbal pastes on the thyroid gland are adviced. Internal medications are prescribed as well.

Yoga

Yoga asanas like Matsyasana, Sarvangasana, Halasana, Viparita Karani, and Pawanmuktasana are suggested along with pranayamas like Brahmari, Ujjayi, and Nadi Shodhana.

Skin Rashes

Skin rashes could occur due to various reasons. The appearance of such rashes could be different too. They can appear as tiny little eruptions, mostly reddish, in crops anywhere on the body. They present mostly along with itchiness. They could be dry or might be wet from scratching. Gradually, most of it spreads to form a larger patch. Over a period of time, these rashes turn darker and sometimes thicker, with extreme dryness and itchiness.

They appear mostly on limbs and around the neck and upper back. Rarely are they seen on the abdomen or face.

If proper care is not taken, these rashes could turn eczematous.

Causes

Skin rashes appear as a result of bites from insects, allergies to clothes, perfume, cosmetics etc, allergies to food or pollutants, allergies to some internal medications, or simply as the body's reaction to the toxins within oneself. Rashes appear also as a result of stress.

Prevention

- Drinking ample water (2–3 litres) per day is the first step towards detoxification. It also keeps the skin hydrated and reduces the intensity of the rashes.
- Try to analyze the cause, and avoid it totally.
- Allergies if any should be specially treated and avoided.
- Never use hot water to bathe, as it dehydrates the skin. Dryness leads to itchyness.
- Always wear clean cotton garments to enable the skin to breathe easily.
- Open and fresh air helps the skin breathe better.
- Try and avoid scratching, as it may lead to super invaded infections.
- Be gentle in handling your skin; use gentle moisturizers, soap etc.
- Always use a moisturizer on the skin. It could be pure coconut oil or olive oil mixed with almond oil and should be applied immediately after bathing. This locks in moisture.

Holistic approach

The approach to skin according to the holistic view starts from the mind. Emotional stress and tensions have a lot of influence on skin conditions. So the approach definitely involves balancing the mind through various treatments, deep breathing, pranayamas, and meditation.

Diet too plays a great role. Simply following a vegetarian diet cooked with low salt and spices and drinking lot of water etc. can heal the skin. Digestive disturbances like acidity and constipation are eliminated through diet and medications.

Internal medications and treatments help to improve skin conditions and prevent further infection.

Homeopathy

Rhus Tox can be given for simple allergic rashes with a lot of itching. Belladona is a good medicine for skin rashes due to sun sensitivity. Kali Mur 6x acts as a skin tonic and can be taken for general skin conditions. Major skin conditions like eczema, psoriasis, and lichen planus need to be evaluated by a homeopathic doctor and treated holistically.

Naturopathy

- Epsom salt (Magnesium Sulphate) acts as a mild skin irritant and helps reduce itchiness.
- Epsom salt can be made into a paste with water and applied directly on the rashes.
- Organic turmeric powder mixed with neem oil helps the condition.
- Neem leaves, ground with turmeric into a fine paste, can be applied to reduce the itchiness and also dry up the rashes.
- Boil water with neem leaves, fresh crushed turmeric and Epsom salt. Fill it in a tub, and make the person lie in it to reduce the rashes and itchiness.
- Food intake should be regulated too. Meals should include fruits and vegetables.
- It's better to avoid carbohydrates, milk and its products, junk food, spicy food and oily food, and nuts for a few days to enable detoxification.
- Take fruit and vegetable juices and dry fruits in plenty.
- Fasting therapy is advised where one refrains from cooked food. Either only liquids or fruits are given to ensure complete detoxification.
- Yogic techniques help to strengthen the skin through physical, mental and spiritual levels.

Ayurveda

Ayurveda believes the root cause for rashes to be impure blood. So detoxification is the key. Ayurveda believes in the treatment of the actual cause of the disease be it the allergies or stress, rather than the rashes per se.

- External applications like Eladi Choornam with coconut milk and Eladi Thailam, Nalpamaradi Thailam are helpful in preventing dryness and itchiness and to moisturize the skin.
- Paste of Durva(Cynodon Dactylon) with turmeric is used for external application.
- In children, Chembaruthiyadi Tailam is used.
- Bathing with Nalpamara Kashayam, water boiled with Durva and turmeric etc. help.
- Avoid using soap. Paste made of green gram flour, turmeric and curd could be used instead.
- Aloe vera pulp could be used on the skin to prevent itchiness.

Migraines

The word migraine is derived from the Greek word Hemi Crania which mean 'pain on one side of the head'. Migraine headaches tend to first appear between the ages of 10 and 45. Sometimes they may begin later in life. Migraines are about three times more common in women than in men and may run in families. Some women, but not all, may have fewer migraines when they are pregnant.

A migraine is a common type of headache that may occur with symptoms such as nausea, vomiting, or sensitivity to light. In many people, a throbbing pain is felt only on one side of the head. Some people who get migraines have warning symptoms called an aura, before the actual headache begins. An aura is a group of symptoms, including vision disturbances, that are a warning that a bad headache is coming.

Causes

Alcohol, stress and anxiety, certain odours or perfumes, loud noises or bright lights, and smoking may trigger a migraine. Migraine attacks may also be triggered by caffeine withdrawal, changes in hormone levels during a woman's menstrual cycle, or with the use of birth control pills. Changes in sleep patterns, exercise or other physical stress, missed meals, smoking, or exposure to smoke can also cause the headaches.

Common symptoms

A typical migraine headache is unilateral, throbbing, moderate to severe, and can be aggravated by physical activity. Not all these symptoms are necessary. The pain may be bilateral at the onset or start on one side and become generalized, and may occur primarily on one side or alternate sides from one attack to the next. The onset is usually gradual. The pain peaks and then subsides and usually lasts for 2–72 hours in adults and 1–48 hours in children. The frequency of attacks is extremely variable, from a few in a lifetime to several a week, and the average sufferer experiences one to three headaches a month. The head pain varies greatly in intensity, and can be very severe.

Prevention

Preventive treatments of migraines include medications, nutritional supplements, and lifestyle alterations. The goal is to reduce the frequency, painfulness, and/or duration of migraines.

Lifestyle changes can reduce the frequency of migraine attacks and make a difference in your migraines.

- Avoid or limit triggers.
- Wake up and go to bed the same time every day.
- Eat healthy foods and do not skip meals.
- Engage in regular physical activity.
- Limit alcohol and caffeine intake.
- Learn ways to reduce and cope with stress.

Holistic approach

This approach focuses on treatments for the stress and to strengthen the nervous system etc. depending on the causative factors. Herbal remedies, homeopathy remedies, and special ayurvedic therapies help to detoxify the body and help in rejuvenation. Aromatherapy, acupuncture, acupressure, reflexology, enema, hydrotherapy, and therapeutic diet have been very beneficial in the treatment of migraines as well. Yoga therapy with breathing techniques, deep relaxation, and meditation techniques plays an important role in prevention and treatment of migraine.

Homeopathy

Belladona is given for right sided headaches with eye pains and photosensitivity. Gelsemium is for headaches from exposure to sun and tension. Sanguinaria is a good medicine for right sided headaches and Spigelia for left sided headaches. Iris Versicolour works well for migraine headaches associated with vomiting and nausea. In homeopathy the recurrent episodes of migraine can be prevented by treating the root cause which is evaluated by a homeopathic practitioner.

Naturopathy

The attempt is to try to decongest the crania and to relax the nerves through treatments like arm and foot baths, spinal baths, mud applications to the head and neck etc. Following a low-spice, low-fat diet helps a lot in reducing the frequency and intensity of the attacks. Avoiding sugar, foods with preservatives, flavouring agents, and colouring agents also helps overcome the symptoms. One should drink lot of water, as dehydration can trigger severe attacks.

Acupuncture is the most effective method in treating migraines. Specific points on the scalp, neck and hands are stimulated which act instantly and also give long- term benefits.

Ayurveda

Depending on the predominant dosha, medicated oil, buttermilk, or milk is used for Dhara. Thalam with herbal pastes, external application of Kachuram paste on the forehead, application of dry ginger with curd etc. are done. Nasya, Virechanam, and Vasti help too. Warm light food, not too oily, which is easily digestible should be taken. Internal medications like Varanadi Kashayam and Pathyashadangam are prescribed.

Yoga

Yogic kriya Jalaneti, and eye wash help the condition. Pranayamas like Nadi Shodhana, Brahmari, Seetali and Seetkari are suggested. Yoga Nidra and deep relaxation techniques help a lot.

Kitchen cures

❖ Massaging the forehead with primrose oil is beneficial in curing migraines.

❖ Cabbage leaves are helpful in relieving the pain of a migraine headache. Squash cabbage leaves and place them in a cloth. Place the cloth on your forehead for some time. Once the cabbage leaves become dry, remove the cloth and make a fresh one.

- Lemon peel is helpful in the headache too. Grind lemon peel to form a paste and apply it on the forehead. Let it dry and then rinse off with cool water.
- A mixture of carrot juice, either with spinach, beet or cucumber juice, works effectively in curing migraines. Combine 300 ml of carrot juice with 200 ml of any other juice and drink it.
- Chew 2 tsp of cumin seeds with jaggery (palm sugar) and then drink a glass of warm water. This helps to reduce the headache.

Dark Circles

Dark circles are dark blemishes around the eyes. Dark circles under eyes usually are a sign of exhaustion, though they can make you feel old, unhealthy, and tired. Dark circles under eyes affect both men and women, often starting in adulthood, although children can develop dark circles under eyes, too.

Dark circles are likely to become more noticeable and permanent with age. This is because as people get older, their skin loses collagen, becoming thinner and more translucent.

Causes

Lack of sleep or excessive tiredness can cause paleness of the skin, allowing the blood underneath to become more visible and appear bluer or darker. Lack of nutrients in your diet, or the lack of a balanced diet, can contribute to the discolouration of the area under the eyes. It is believed that lack of mineral iron can cause dark circles as well. Iron deficiency is the most common type of anaemia and this condition is a sign that not enough oxygen is getting to the body tissues. Any condition that causes the eyes to itch can contribute to darker circles due to rubbing or scratching of the skin around them. Some food allergies can also cause the area under the eyes to appear darker.

However, dark under-eye circles usually aren't a medical problem, and home remedies for dark circles under eyes may be all you need to help manage this condition.

Prevention

- Appropriate treatment of allergies, nasal congestions, and other medical conditions.
- Adequate fluid intake.
- Avoid smoking, excessive salt intake and sun exposure.
- Eating foods rich in Vitamin C. These include cranberries, blueberries, bilberries, tea (green or black), black currants, onions, legumes, and parsley, and dietary supplements such as grape seed extracts.

Holistic approach

Holistic approach in reducing dark under eye circles basically involves all aspects of a person's life. Therapies like special ayurvedic facials, fruit and vegetable facials, massage with herbal oils, mud packs are beneficial. All of them will help to tone the skin and reduce the circles under your eyes.

Homeopathy

Dark circles can be hereditary or they can also develop due to stress, tiredness, sleeplessness, or long hours in front of computers. A constitutional approach helps in reducing the dark circles. Application of Berberis Aquifolium around the eyes will reduce the dark circles.

Naturopathy

Mud packs or cold packs to the eyes, eye washes with rose water, washing the eyes with water stored in copper vessel or tulsi etc. help relax the eyes and prevent dark circles.

Ayurveda
Depending on the root cause, treatments to de-stress and improve the quality of sleep, to reduce fatigue and to nourish the body are done. Special herbal oil applications like Kumkumadi Tailam, Nalpamaradi Tailam, and virgin coconut oil also help. Apply a paste of red sandal, curd and turmeric.

Yoga
Yoga improves blood circulation, tones muscles and skin, reduces stress levels, and improves the oxygen concentration in the blood thereby reducing dark circles.

Deep relaxation techniques like Yoga Nidra give adequate rest and relaxation. Pranayamas are particularly beneficial inimproving oxygenation to the cells of the skin, thereby reducing dark circles and improving skin tone.

Kitchen cures
Mild to moderate dark circles often respond well to simple treatments, such as the following:

- Try a cold compress of two chilled teaspoons or a bag of frozen peas wrapped in a soft cloth to temporarily reduce dilated and discoloured under-eye blood vessels. Or use a cooled teabag.
- Apply cool cucumber slices over closed eyes for 15 minutes.
- Elevate your head with two or more pillows to prevent puffiness that develops when fluid pools in your lower eyelids.
- Lack of sleep makes you paler and more hollow-eyed, so shadows and circles you already have become more obvious.
- Rinsing your sinuses with a saltwater solution (mix ¼ teaspoon sea salt with 2 cups of warm water).
- Mix fresh potato juice and cucumber juice in equal amounts. Soak some cotton in the above mixture and put

on your eyelids for 20 minutes. Wash off with cold water.

- One can use rose water or almond oil for massaging the under eyes dark circle, to get rid of them.
- Grind nutmeg with milk and make a paste. Apply this paste on the dark circles. Make a paste blending tomatoes and lemon juice in equal amounts. Add a pinch of gram flour and turmeric powder, apply the paste and leave it for 15 minutes. This will do wonders in curing dark circles.

DR MATHAI'S TIPS

- Harmful rays of the sun can also cause eye circles. Hence you should wear sunglasses while going out.
- Stress is, yet again, one of the major causes for dark circles under the eyes. If you are under a lot of stress, it will show on your face. Breathing exercises and meditation help to keep out the stress.

Sleeplessness

Insomnia is a common problem that takes a toll on your energy, mood, health and ability to function during the day. Chronic insomnia can even contribute to serious health problems. But simple changes to your lifestyle and daily habits can mostly put a stop to sleepless nights.

Insomnia is the inability to get the amount of sleep you need, to wake up feeling rested and refreshed. Because different people need different amounts of sleep, insomnia is defined by the quality of your sleep and how you feel after sleeping—not the number of hours you sleep or how quickly you doze off. Even if you're spending eight hours a night in bed, and you feel drowsy and fatigued during the day, you may be experiencing insomnia.

Although insomnia is the most common sleep complaint, it is not a singular sleep disorder. It is more accurate to think of insomnia as a symptom of another problem. The problem causing the insomnia differs from person to person. It could be something as simple as drinking too much caffeine during the day or a more complex issue like an underlying medical condition or feeling overloaded with responsibilities.

The good news is that most cases of insomnia can be cured with changes you can make on your own without relying on sleep specialists or turning to prescription or over-the-counter sleeping pills.

Causes

In order to properly treat and cure your insomnia, you need to become a sleep detective. Emotional issues such as stress, anxiety, and depression cause half of all insomnia cases. But your daytime habits, sleep routine and physical health may also play a role. Try to identify all possible causes for your insomnia. Once you figure out the root cause, you can tailor treatment accordingly.

- Are you under a lot of stress?
- Are you depressed? Do you feel emotionally flat or hopeless?
- Do you struggle with chronic feelings of anxiety or worry?
- Have you recently gone through a traumatic experience?
- Are you taking any medications that might be affecting your sleep?
- Do you have any health problems that may be interfering with sleep?
- Is your sleep environment quiet and comfortable?
- Are you spending enough time in sunlight during the day and in darkness at night?
- Do you try to go to bed and get up around the same time every day?

Common mental and physical causes of insomnia:
Sometimes, insomnia only lasts a few days and goes away on its own, especially when the insomnia is tied to an obvious temporary cause, such as stress over an upcoming presentation, a painful breakup, or jet lag. Other times, insomnia is stubbornly persistent. Chronic insomnia is usually tied to an underlying mental or physical issue.

- **Psychological problems that can cause insomnia:** Depression, anxiety, chronic stress, bipolar disorder, post-traumatic stress disorder.
- **Medications that can cause insomnia:** Antidepressants; cold and flu medications that contain alcohol; pain relievers that contain caffeine (Midol, Excedrin); diuretics, corticosteroids, thyroid hormone, high blood pressure medications.
- **Medical problems that can cause insomnia:** Asthma, allergies, Parkinson's disease, hyperthyroidism, acid reflux, kidney disease, cancer, or chronic pain.
- **Sleep disorders that can cause insomnia:** Sleep apnea, narcolepsy, restless legs syndrome.

Most people suffering from an anxiety disorder or depression have trouble sleeping. What's more, the sleep deprivation can make the symptoms of anxiety or depression worse. If your insomnia is caused by anxiety or depression, treating the underlying psychological issue is the key to the cure.

Prevention

- Make sure your bedroom is quiet, dark, and cool. Noise, light, and heat can interfere with sleep. Try using a sound machine or earplugs to mask outside noise, an open window or fan to keep the room cool, and blackout curtains or an eye mask to block out light.

- Stick to a regular sleep schedule. Support your biological clock by going to bed and getting up at the same time every day, including weekends. Get up at your usual time in the morning even if you're tired. This will help you get back in a regular sleep rhythm.
- Avoid naps. Napping during the day can make it more difficult to sleep at night. If you feel like you have to take a nap, limit it to 30 minutes before 3 pm.
- Avoid stimulating activity and stressful situations before bedtime. This includes vigorous exercise; big discussions or arguments; and TV, computer, or video game use.
- Limit caffeine, alcohol, and nicotine. Stop drinking caffeinated beverages at least 8 hours before bed. Avoid drinking in the evening. While alcohol can make you feel sleepy, it interferes with the quality of your sleep. Quit smoking or avoid it at night, as nicotine is a stimulant.

Holistic approach

Sleeplessness can be very well treated with a holistic approach. Ayurvedic therapies like Sirodhara, Takradhara, Shirolepam, Thalam, Abhyanga Nasyam help to improve circulation, condition the subconscious mind and thus improve the quality of sleep. Therapeutic diet also plays an important role in such a condition. Drinking warm sweet drinks at bed time induce good sleep eg. warm water or milk with honey. Yoga therapies with specific asanas, breathing techniques, and relaxation and meditation techniques relaxe the mind and induce quality sleep. This would include pranayamas like Brahmari and Ujjayi, Yoga Nidra, and Shavasana.

Homeopathy

Passiflora Q in water at night helps in good sleep. Kali Phos soothes the nerves and helps too. Nux Vomica also helps in sleep especially for people who are very agitated. For sleeplessness, often homeopathic constitutional approach is taken.

Naturopathy

- Simple measures like lighting the bedroom with blue coloured light can induce good sleep.
- Taking a hot shower before going to bed also helps.
- Taking a hot foot bath by immersing your feet and calves into hot water can be helpful.

Ayurveda

Sleeplessness in ayurveda is because of the disturbance in the Vata and Pitta. Insomnia in turn disturbs Vata and forms a vicious cycle. So treatments to pacify Vata and Pitta like Sirodhara, Abhyanga, Thalam, Takradhara, and general detoxification are all helpful. A nourishing diet with milk and ghee is also helpful.

Herbs like Aswagandha, Brahmi, and Vidari are good solutions as well.

YOGASANAS FOR VARIOUS CONDITIONS

	CONDITION	RECOMMENDED YOGASANA
1	Hypothyroidsm	1. Head, neck, and shoulder excercises 2. Asanas: Makarabyasa, Setubandhasana 3. Pranayama: Nadi Shudhi and Brahmari 4. Relaxation techniques
2	Diabetes	1. Head-to-toe loosening exercises 2. Asanas: Padahastasana, Ardha Chakrasana, Parswa Chakrasana, Ustrasana, Vakrasana, Makarabyasa 3. Pranayama: Chandra Nadi and Nadi Shudhi. 4. Relaxation techniques
3	Hypertension	1. Head-to-toe loosening exercises 2. Asanas: Tadasana, Vakrasana, Makarabyasa 3. Pranayama: Chandra Nadi, Brahmari 4. Relaxation and Meditation techniques
4	Arthritis	1. Head-to-toe loosening exercises 2. Pranayama: Nadi Shudhi and Brahmari 3. Relaxation techniques
5	Bone health	1. Asanas: Tadasana, Padahastasana, Ardha Chakrasana, Parswa Chakrasana, Vikrasana, Ustrasana, Makarabhayasa, Setubandhasana, Bhujangasana, Salabhasana 2. Pranayama: Nadi Shudhi 3. Relaxation and Meditation techniques
6	Constipation	1. Asanas: Tadasana, Padahastasana, Ardha Chakrasana, Parswa Chakrasana, Vikrasana, Ustrasana, Makarabhayasa, Setubandhasana, Bhujangasana, Salabhasana 2. Pranayama: Bhastrika 3. Relaxation techniques
7	Hair health	General yogasanas and relaxation techniques
8	Skin health	General yogasanas and relaxation techniques

	CONDITION	RECOMMENDED YOGASANA
9	Obesity	1. Suryanamaskar, 12 rounds 2. Asanas: Tadasana, Padahastasana, Ardha Chakrasana, Parswa Chakrasana, Vikrasana, Ustrasana, Makarabhayasa, Setubandhasana, Bhujangasana, Salabhasana 3. Pranayama: Nadi Shudhi 4. Relaxation and Meditation techniques
10	Headache/ migraine	1. Yoga Kriyas 2. Pranayama: Chandra Nadi, Brahmari, and Nadi Shudhi 3. Relaxation and Meditation techniques

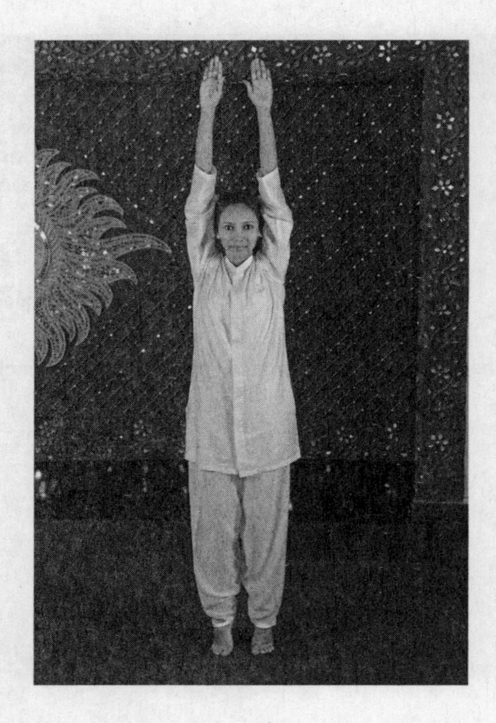

Tadasana (palm tree pose)

- Stand straight with your legs together.
- With inhalation, raise the arms and simultaneously the heels up.
- Stretch the entire body.
- Fix the gaze on a point for better sense of balance.
- Breath in and out normally and hold the posture comfortably, feeling the stretch in the entire spine, ankles and shoulders.
- With an exhalation slowly lower the hands and place the heels on the ground.
- Relax completely.

Benefits

Tadasana improves the sense of balance

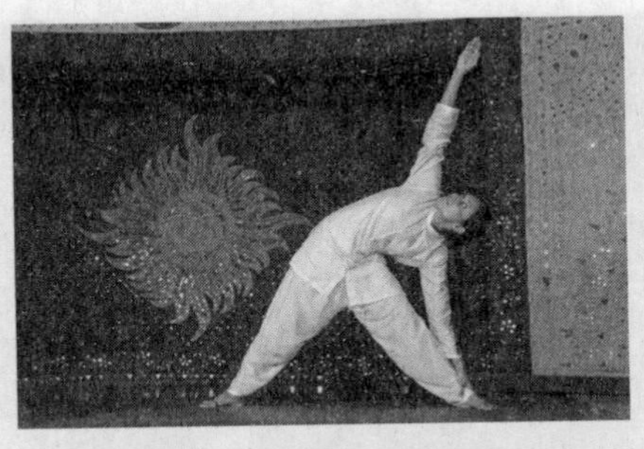

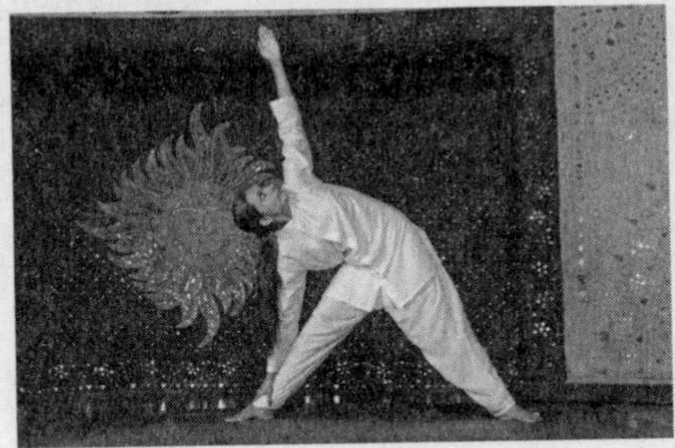

Trikonasana (triangle pose)

- Stand with the legs wide apart, more than the shoulder distance.
- Inhale and raise the arms up to the shoulder level, sideways.
- With an exhalation, tilt to the right side, making sure not to move the body forward.
- Try to hold the right ankle with the right hand.
- The left arm is extended upwards with the fingers pointing up.
- Turn the head and look up at the left hand which is above.
- If needed you can bend the right knee slightly. The left knee is straight.
- Feel the stretch on the sides of the body.
- With an inhalation, straighten the spine and knee.
- Exhale and bring the hands down.
- Relax.
- Repeat on the other side, by tilting to the left and looking up at the right hand.

Benefits

This posture tones the pelvic organs, strengthens the reproductive system and eliminates the excess fat from the waist line

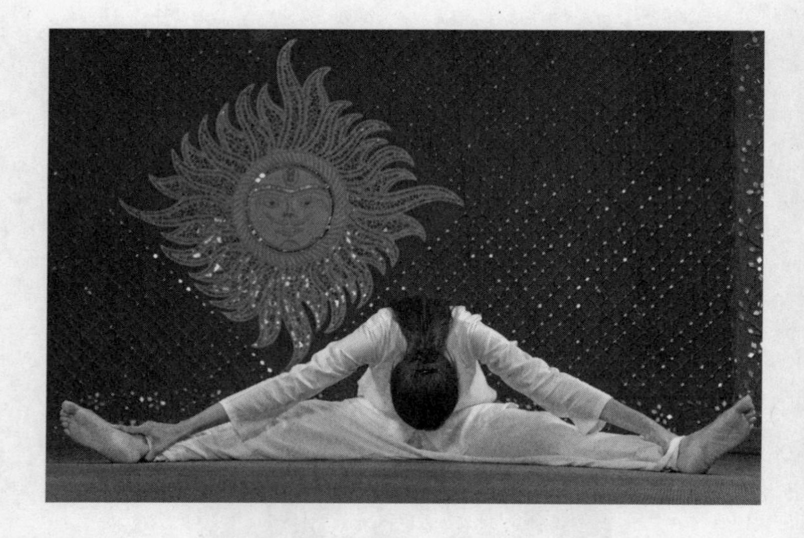

Upavista Konasana

- Sit with your legs stretched out.
- Now slowly move the legs apart to your sides, as far as you can go.
- Do not lift your knees up.
- With an exhalation, slowly bend forward, as much as possible.
- Hands should be placed on the legs.
- If possible without hurting the back, one should try to touch the chin to the floor.
- If not, hold where ever possible comfortably.
- Do not over stretch, as this may cause injury to the ligaments.
- With an inhalation slowly straighten the spine and relax.

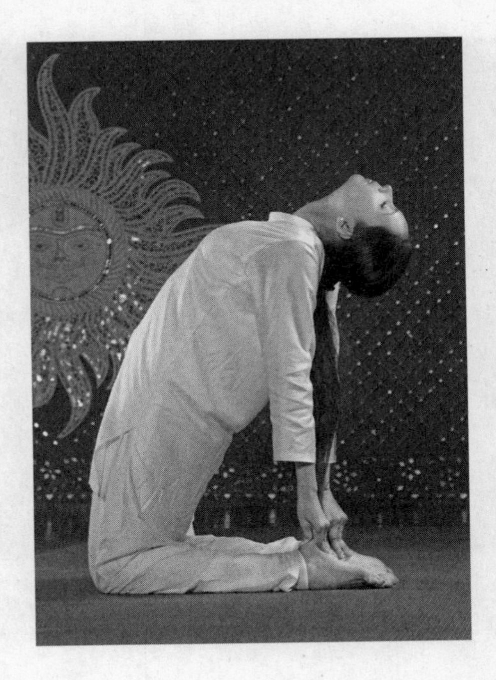

Ustrasana (camel pose)

- Stand on the knees, either placed together or slightly apart.
- Place the hands on the respective hip.
- Inhale and bend back as much as you can.
- Let the shoulders and neck be relaxed.
- Feel the compression in the entire spine while you continue normal breathing.
- If possible try to release the hands and hold the ankle with the respective hand.
- With an exhalation, straighten the spine and sit down with the legs stretched comfortably.
- Lie on the abdomen with the legs stretched.

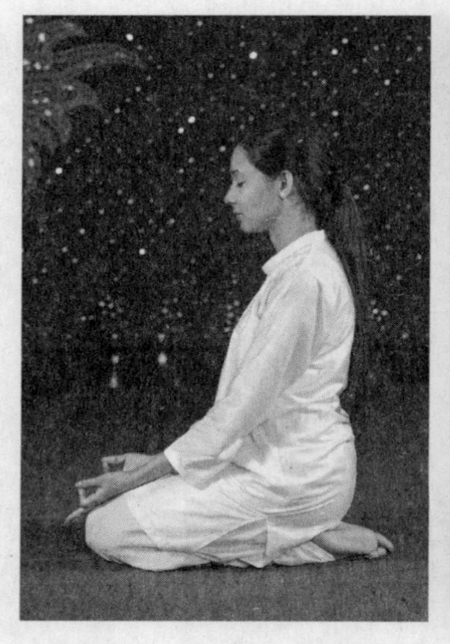

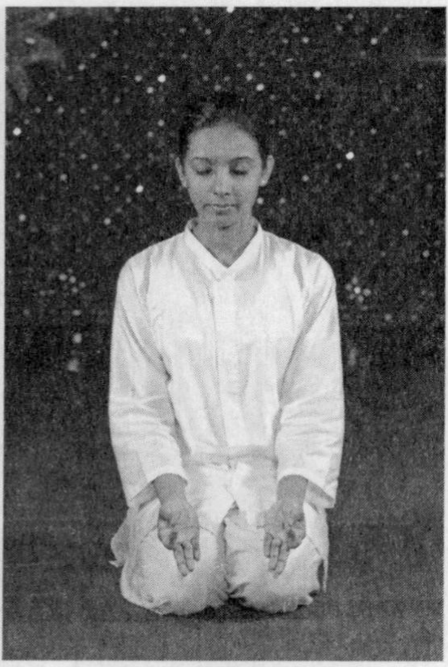

Vajrasana

- This is a sitting posture.
- Bend the right leg at the knee and place the right buttock on the right heel.
- Now bend the left knee and place the left buttock on the left heel.
- Place the heels such that the great toes touch each other.
- You are now comfortably sitting on the heels.
- Hands could just rest on the knees or thighs with the palms facing up or down.
- One could also place them in 'chin' mudra, that is the thumb touching the index finger and the rest of the fingers opened out.

Benefits

Vajrasana is a meditative posture • This is the only asana you could practice immediately after a meal • It's adviced to sit in vajrasana for 10 minutes prior and 10 minutes after a meal • The circulation is drawn towards the digestive system • It regularizes blood sugar and hence is best advised in diabetes • You can feel the stretch in the ankles and thighs

Part III

Lifestyle Conditions

AROUND THE AGE OF FORTY-FIVE OR THE MENOPAUSAL stage of your life, you may begin to notice early signs of ageing as manifested in the onset of hereditary and lifestyle symptoms like stress and grey hair. It is important not to accept these in a fatalistic surrender of control. I have noticed in several cases, patients attribute their symptoms to 'growing old' and surrender themselves to fate without even trying to take on the challenge of changing their lifestyles or questioning signs of ill-health. It is imperative that as soon as you notice any early signs (eg. of arthritis), that you have a proper medical assessment done and do not ignore potential health issues.

At this important stage in your life, you must be conscious of your eating patterns, your exercise routine, and other lifestyle-related behaviours (drinking, smoking, sleep patterns). I would advise you not to use over-the-counter, stop-gap measures to deal with any symptoms. For instance, an aspirin to relieve chronic pain is not ideal when there could possibly be an underlying reason for it. Routine and annual medical checkups become a must in maintaining a healthy lifestyle. I would like to emphasize that timely intervention can help prevent lifestyle related chronic conditions.

At the elderly stage, once again, continuing to go on with life as it was earlier is of the utmost importance. If a woman gives in to her age, withdrawing from activities and exercise, she will invariably develop some condition or other that will prevent her from participating in the daily activities of her life. I would like to stress that at this stage in life, you need not give up an active lifestyle. Exercise—though less vigorous, perhaps—is still important to keep the body functioning at its best. Diet, social activities, and just doing things for yourself are all important factors in this stage your life.

Our lifestyle defines us. It is the way we live our lives, what we do, with whom, and where. Our lifestyle encompasses everything—from the food we eat to how we interact with people around us to even the way we get around. Our lifestyle has changed dramatically over the last few years. We are more sedentary than before. We have machines to do our work for us. We have vehicles for our travel. We are more dependent on assisted movement than our own bodies. Increased consumption of unhealthy food and fast food to save time is the norm. The environment has become more polluted due to increased vehicular traffic. Life is more hectic for most people with less time to relax. Now there is also an increased exposure to electronic stimulation via mobile, television etc. People are more prone to stress at work and in personal life so they don't take care of the rhythms in their life. Children do not play anymore as they have no space to play or are glued to TV or video games.

While many of the above points may seem to be inevitable, these are causing constant stress on our body and mind without our knowledge. Coping with day-to-day stress is necessary to lead a long and healthy life. There are few steps that can be taken to cope with these:

- Exercise regularly.
- Eat healthy and organic food.
- Cook most of your meals at home and carry food to work.
- Travel short distances by walking or cycling.
- Relax for sometime in a day by doing nothing or just being in a garden.
- Maintain the rhythm in your life with regards to eating time, sleeping time, and exercise time.
- Spend some time with yourself, preferably in the morning, to reflect and plan the day.

Taking care of one's health is the responsibility of each individual. We have to be responsible for our health and well being for no one else will be. Certain precautions and actions can help us in this task and we should follow them diligiously.

- Maintain a regular schedule for eating and sleeping. In this way, you will maintain the rhythm of your life too.
- Exercise regularly for a fixed period of time. Include both stretching and cardio in the workout regimen.
- Eat healthy food.
- Include lot of vegetables and fruits in your diet.
- Add variety to your food.
- Adopt healthy cooking habits.
- Avoid alcohol, smoking, chewing ghutka etc.
- Manage stress. Take professional help when you feel you are not able to cope.

CHAPTER NINE

Stress

Why do Women Get Stressed?

Women frequently carry out multiple roles including those of a professional, a mom, a spouse, a caregiver and so on. It can be exciting to have many responsibilities, but multi-tasking can become overly demanding and almost impossible to handle sometimes. Women tend to feel overwhelmed by this role overload and may end up feeling burned out. Women often tend to give to others at the expense of themselves. They frequently spend most of their physical and emotional energy on family, work, and their household, while neglecting themselves almost completely. Many women feel selfish if they focus on their own physical and emotional needs. Women also tend to be perfectionists and create self-imposed stress with the high expectations they have for themselves.

Hormonal changes in a woman's body can increase a female's vulnerability to feelings of stress. This can vary with hormone levels throughout a monthly menstrual cycle and throughout the stages of life. Women may experience a heightened susceptibility to stress post-delivery as well. Those undergoing menopause may experience varying levels of stress or mood changes.

Common symptoms

- ❖ Symptoms of stress include feeling tense, depressed, or angry.
- ❖ Having difficulty in making decisions.
- ❖ Frequent mood swings, negative thinking.
- ❖ Excess smoking, drinking or eating.
- ❖ Feeling overwhelmed or helpless.

Stress is an expression of the body's natural instinct to protect itself. But prolonged stress can have negative effect the physical and emotional health.

Chronic stress increases the risks for a number of conditions including backaches, high blood pressure, thyroid disorders, sexual dysfunction, ulcers, headaches, and weight gain. Other physical risks include skin disorders, eating disorders, emotional upsets, arthritis, immune disorders, cancer, and sleep problem.

Holistic approach

- ❖ Set aside relaxation time.
- ❖ Get adequate sleep and sleep on a regular schedule.
- ❖ Take time to eat a nutritious meal.
- ❖ Exercise regularly. This can reduce the risk of several stress related conditions.
- ❖ Limit watching TV or using computer and the internet.
- ❖ Take time to reflect on life. Take help, if needed.
- ❖ Manage your time well and eliminate unnecessary tasks.
- ❖ Keep in touch with friends and have occasional get togethers.
- ❖ Stay organized.
- ❖ Good communication with life partner, family members and friends.

Do-it-yourself routines

- Take time for yourself everyday. This can be 15 minutes to an hour or more. Do your favourite activity during this time like singing, playing a musical instrument, gardening, and painting.
- Practice deep breathing/Pranayama daily for 15–30 minutes.
- Have a journal to write down the day activities and interactions at the end of the day before going to sleep.

Symptoms of stress

1. Acne

Acne usually starts at adolescence. It's a condition where the skin shows eruptions especially on the face, though it could affect the neck and upper back.

It develops as rashes, sometimes reddish with white tips or heads. It could be solitary or in crops. It could turn very painful and the size varies. It could leave scars especially if frequently touched or picked by hands. It could also get infected. The whiteheads could eventually turn black.

Acne occurs as a result of overactive sebaceous glands. The role of sebum is to keep the skin moisturized. It's an oily secretion. This when secreted in excess, and when not cleaned properly, clogs the skin giving rise to acne. Over secretion of sebum occurs during adolescence due to the hormonal changes. Dandruff, oily food, junk food, constipation, stress, irregular menstruation, obesity, lack of hygiene, and regular skin care are all contributing factors. Hormonal disorders like PCOS, hypothyroidism, and high testosterone secretion are also contributing factors.

Prevention

- Wash your face at least twice a day with mild soap or a herbal product.
- Take care of dandruff, with regular shampooing and use medications if needed.
- Avoid junk food and deep fried food.
- Include lots of water, fresh vegetables and fruits, and fibre in the diet.
- Exercise regularly to let the skin breathe better, to improve the circulation to the skin, and to open up the pores.
- Do not touch the eruptions or pick at them.
- Avoid constipation.

Holistic approach

When we look at acne from a holistic view point, we need to consider the genetic factors, the mental status of the individual prior and post its occurrence, the involvement of the various organs and systems and their functions.

First of all we try to find the cause through a holistic evaluation. The treatments would focus on detoxification of the system, thereby improving digestion, relieving constipation etc. If any hormonal abnormalities are found, we correct that through treatments and internal medications. We try to analyse her food habits and lifestyle and help her make necessary changes.

General counselling is done to help her overcome the embarrassment and difficulty in facing people.

Contributing factors like dandruff are taken care of through proper treatments.

Internal medications to continue are prescribed along with diet and yoga and simple steps or treatments which could be done at home.

The treatments done at the centre would include Sirodhara, Abhyanga, herbal packs, and mud treatments.

Homeopathy

Kali Brom can be taken twice a day to reduce pimples. Berberis Aquifolium Q application on the face can reduce acne. Acne can be due to stomach issues and then Nux Vomica is a good remedy. Adult acne can be caused due to hormonal changes. This needs to be investigated and a proper homeopathic evaluation needs to be made.

Naturopathy

- Wash your face regularly with green gram flour mixed with turmeric powder and raw milk.
- Steam on the face, from water boiled with tulsi and neem leaves.
- Apply a paste of tender guava leaves/neem leaves/mint leaves and turmeric and wash it off after 20 minutes.
- A paste made of fuller's earth and curd could be applied too.
- Mashed pulp of fruits such as papaya and banana helps.

Ayurveda

The approach is to treat the underlying cause through proper medications. Detoxification plays a major role, especially Virechanam with appropriate herbs.

- Internal medications are important too.
- External applications like Eladi Choornam with milk helps to heal acne and prevent scars.
- To reduce the pain, cinnamon powder mixed with water can be applied externally.
- Paste of red sandal mixed with Kasturi Manjal helps to prevent scars.
- Mint leaves and turmeric paste helps to cleanse the skin.
- If this leads to depression, then that aspect should be treated appropriately.

Yoga

Yoga plays an important role in regulating the hormones, improving circulation to the skin, calming the mind, and improving overall health.

2. Hair Loss

Hair loss could mean either loss from the head or from the body. This includes variety of reasons such as environmental, nutritional, genetic, or due to some infection.

Causes

- Diabetes.
- Fungal infections.
- Hair treatments (chemicals in relaxers, hair straighteners).
- Hereditary disorders.
- Hormonal changes.
- Hyperthyroidism and hypothyroidism.
- Iron deficiency or malnutrition in general.
- Medications (side effects from drugs, including chemotherapy, anabolic steroids, and birth control pills).
- Scalp infection.
- Secondary syphilis.
- Stress.

Holistic approach

Natural and holistic treatments are a gentler and effective alternative to treating hair loss than the harsh chemicals. Using herbal and homeopathic remedies helps to promote healthy strong hair and supports circulation, hormonal balance and thyroid functioning. It is advisable to wash your hair daily or alternate days using herbal shampoo or any baby shampoo diluted with water. Contributing factors like dandruff etc. are taken care of through proper treatments.

Ayurveda

Ayurvedic herbal hair oils like Neelibringadi Tailam, Kayyunyadi Tailam etc. are helpful in hair growth depending on the condition.

Diet

- Melons, berries, bananas, oranges, apples, and many other fruits can supply your body with the proper vitamins to reduce hair loss.
- While all vegetables will provide your hair with additional vitamins, the ones that offer the most benefits are those of the green leafy variety, including spinach and cabbage.
- Increasing your dairy intake, including milk, eggs and cheese, can increase your hair's overall health by providing it with Vitamin B-12 as well as protein.
- By adding lean, healthy meats to your diet, or increasing your intake of items like chicken, nuts, fish, and organ meats (such as liver), you will supply your hair follicles with the vitamins they need for optimal operation.
- Consuming at least eight 8 glasses of water per day will help transport the needed nutrients to your hair and help keep your hair strands hydrated and strong.

3. Premature Greying

Premature greying of the hair refers to the greying of hair in the young or before the age of 35 years. Grey hair is caused by gradual reduction of melanin production overtime in your hair follicle. Melanin is the pigment that gives colour and smoothness to your hair. The degree of darkness of your hair depends on how much melanin each hair contains. Eventually, the hair begins to lose its colour and strength when there is less melanin in the hair follicle; the hair becomes dry, brittle, and thinner. Hair loss is also seen sometimes.

Causes

- Improper intake of nutrients in the diet is one of the primary causes of premature greying of hair. Lack of Vitamin B, iron, copper, and iodine in the daily diet are believed to be a contributing factor.
- Prolonged period of stress and anxiety may take a toll on your hair health. It may have an adverse effect on the skin of the scalp, which interferes with the supply of vital nutrition necessary for the health of the hair.
- Heredity: Heredity is one predisposing factor for premature greying. It often runs in the family. In some families, it is noticed that many members develop grey hair at a certain age period, say, as early as in their 20s.
- Unclean condition of scalp weakens the root of the hair as dirt or oils get accumulated in the scalp. It prevents adequate blood supply to the hair shaft through the root to cause premature greying.
- Certain medical conditions like thyroid imbalance, vitiligo, Vitamin B-12 deficiency anaemia etc. are said to be associated with premature greying of hair.

Prevention

There is little you can do to control premature greying if it is a genetically-transmitted disorder. However, you can take some preventive measures to prevent premature greying.

- Diet plays a major role in preventing and arresting premature greying of hair. So, eating lots of fruits and vegetables which contain vitamins and minerals are recommended. Eat dark

green vegetables, yellow fruits, cauliflowers, bananas, and tomatoes. Avoid oily, fried, fatty, and spicy foods.
- Take Vitamin B-12, and pantothenic acid (Vitamin B-5) supplements in your diet. Drink a lot of water.
- Proper grooming of hair is essential to maintain a healthy hair texture and strong roots.
- Use shampoo and conditioners which are mild and suit your hair type.
- Avoid hot water to wash your hair.
- Massage the scalp with your fingertips to ensure proper blood circulation within the scalp.
- Always stay away from using harmful chemicals on your hair like hair colour, hair styling gels etc.
- Exercise regularly to keep the blood well circulated.
- Sleep well to avoid grey hair.

Holistic approach

A holistic evaluation has to be done to analyze the cause of the condition. It is often possible to reverse greying, particularly when it is caused due to an underlying ailment. However, in hereditary cases, greying cannot be reversed but can be effectively controlled.

Homeopathy

Homeopathic medicines are constitutional and individual-specific. They help to control further stretching of grey hair by tackling the underlying cause. Along with the treatment, good dietary guidance is also a must. Internal medications along with diet and yoga and simple steps or treatments can be done at home.

Naturopathy

Head massages followed by Troma packs, if done regularly, can prevent greying.

Ayurveda

Special medicated herbal hair oils are used in ayurveda to prevent and reverse greying. This is used for masssage on the scalp and hair. In certain cases, Sirodhara with these oils is done too.

Some of the oils used are Neelibhringadi, Bhringamalaki, and Kaiyyunyadi.

Kitchen cures

- Boil a few amla (Indian gooseberry) pieces in coconut oil till they turn black. Apply this mixture on your hair to cure premature greying.
- Grate ginger and mix it with a spoon of honey. Eat this mixture everyday.
- Massage coconut oil and lemon juice on your scalp. Boil curry leaves in coconut oil till the leaves become black. Apply on your scalp and hair roots as a hair tonic for hair loss and bringing back the hair pigmentation. Curry leaves contain a natural pigment that helps to retain the natural colour of your hair. Curry leaves can be used with buttermilk or curd to prevent your hair from turning grey.

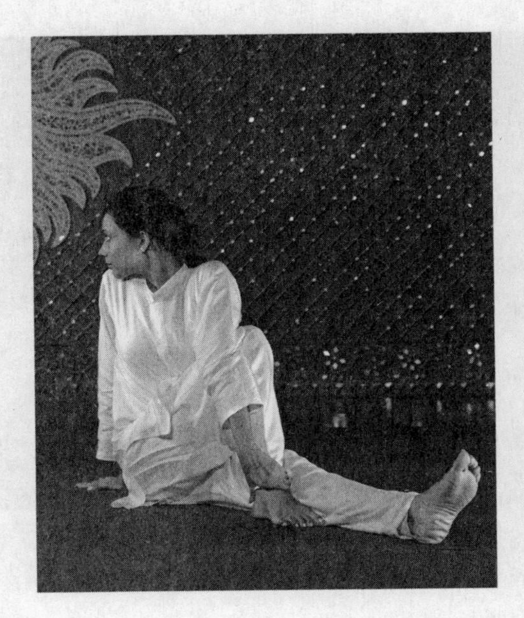

Vakrasana (sitting posture)

- Sit with the legs extended.
- Bend the right leg at the knee, placing the right foot by the side of left inner thigh.
- With an inhalation slowly turn the trunk to the right and place the right palm behind the spine, as close as possible to the spine, such that the spine is straight.
- Hold the right ankle with the left hand.
- With an exhalation turn the head backwards.
- Hold the posture breathing normally.
- With an inhalation turn the head forward, release the right hand, slowly release the left hand and extend the right leg.
- Relax in sitting position and repeat it on the other side.

Benefits

Vakrasana is a spinal twist posture. This posture strengthens the lower back and hips

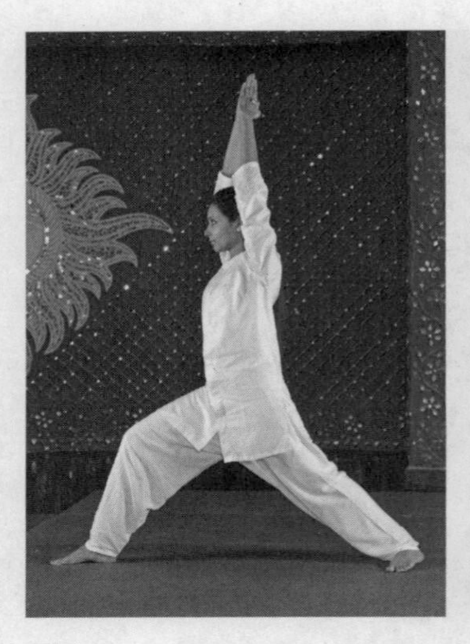

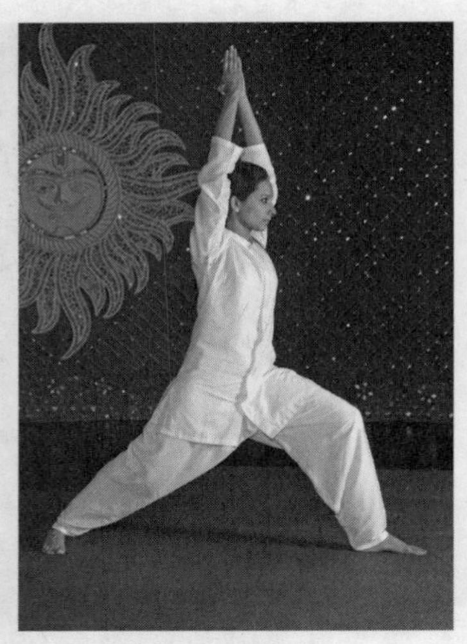

Veerabhadrasana

- Stand with your legs wide apart.
- Bend the right leg at the knee at 90 degrees.
- Turn the right foot to the right, outwards.
- Inhale and raise the arms sideways up to the shoulder level.
- Exhale and turn the trunk to the right.
- Inhale and raise your arms up, above the head and join the palms together in namaskara mudra.
- Breathe normally.
- Left knee should be kept straight.
- You can feel the twist in the spine and the stretch in the shoulders.
- Exhale, bring down the arms to your shoulder level.
- Inhale, turn the spine forward.
- Exhale, bring the arms down, straighten the right knee and turn the foot forward.
- Relax in standing position.
- Repeat on the other side.
- Release and relax.

Benefits

This posture strengthens the knees and the lower limbs

CHAPTER TEN

Ageing

WOMEN ARE AGEING FASTER THAN BEFORE DUE TO THE variety of roles they need to play in their lives, combined with stress, lack of proper and timely nutritious food, lack of exercise and so on. As a result of the hormonal changes that a woman undergoes during the various stages in her life, the signs of ageing are more obvious in her.

Our cells are constantly undergoing change. These cells keep regenerating and replicating themselves continuously, helping us grow. But after a certain age and as a result of food habits, lack of exercise, exposure to toxins and pollutants, emotional and mental stress and the strain of life, this cell regeneration slows down. This slowing down reflects on each and every part in our body, especially the joints, nerves, skin, and hair. These are seen as the signs of ageing.

Before-menopause and Post-menopause Care

The estrogen dip during menopause causes a woman to go through a lot of stress at different levels, hastening the ageing process. Also, hormonal effect on skin, metabolism, hair, and the muscle tone interferes too. So women should take special care of themselves even before the menopause stage is reached.

Prevention

Do-it-yourself tips and what you can do to counter ageing

Following a strict and healthy regime can help you in staying fit, beautiful, healthy, and happy.

- Wake up in the morning with a positive attitude.
- Plan your day.
- Drink 2–3 glasses of water on waking up followed by juice of lemon/vegetables or a cup or two of green tea.
- Exercise for at least 30 minutes—this could be yoga/walking/aerobics/gym.
- Practice meditation and pranayama to keep the mind calm and cheerful.
- Eat a healthy and wholesome breakfast comprising of cereals/bread, fruits, and soaked almonds.
- Include food with lot of fibre like fresh vegetables, fruits, and whole grains in your diet.
- Calcium-rich foods like ragi, oats, green leafy vegetables, and skim milk products should be consumed.
- Include iron-rich foods like dates, black raisins, spinach, and beetroot in your diet.
- Avoid junk food as it could lead to digestive disturbances and weight gain.
- Consume fresh fruits and vegetables in plenty and in raw form along with 8–10 glasses of water per day.
- Make use of the excess vegetables and fruits in the kitchen as skin packs.
- Curd, milk, milk cream, coconut milk, gram flour, turmeric, honey, and lemon could all be used as packs in different combinations.

- Make sure to apply oil on your hair and body, at least 2–3 times a week, before bathing.
- Add lemon juice to the water you bathe in, to remove body odour and to feel fresh.
- Try to use herbal products for body and hair. Find time for your self and engage in your hobbies, listen to good music, read cheerful material, and watch programmes that make you laugh.
- While you watch TV, soak your feet in water with salt to relieve any tiredness.
- Find time to be with friends.
- Make sure you sleep for at least 7 hours.
- Drink a glass of warm skimmed milk before retiring to bed.
- Plan vacations at least twice a year, preferably with friends!
- Indulge in relaxing and pampering treatments like foot spas, facials, and body massages at least once a month.
- Do anti ageing, rejuvenation and detoxification programmes for 15 to 21 days every year.

The saying 'Prevention is better than cure' stands good in the process of ageing. Maintaining a healthy, stress free lifestyle is necessary to delay the ageing process. One should also feel positive in the mind. Regular treatments like massage and relaxation techniques, pampering treatments like facials and reflexology help to de-stress. Avoiding junk food, practicing yogic techniques regularly etc are other things one needs to follow.

Ageing is a slow process and does not happen suddenly. After the most youthful period, generally with the first pregnancy, ageing sets in. If during adolescence, proper care is not taken during one's daily regime, the ageing process hastens. Proper care has to be taken at each stage of a woman's life. This is not only pertaining to the physical self but also the mental and the emotional aspects.

The cell regeneration ceases to happen after certain period. Stress, habits like smoking and alcohol, irregular and inadequate nutrition, lack of exercise, certain illnesses, pollutants, harsh rays of the sun—all of them contribute to the process of ageing.

Having a well-maintained daily regimen involving proper nutritious diet will help delay ageing at the cellular level. Daily exercise involving movements for the body and yogic techniques like breathing, pranayamas, meditation, and relaxation techniques for the mind; indulging in healthy hobbies to stay calm and cheerful; daily skin and haircare regime; avoiding harmful chemical exposure as in cosmetics, using beauty products from nature like milk cream, turmeric, rose water, fruits and vegetables, mud etc are advised. Properly moisturizing the skin and hair with daily application of medicated oil was practiced in households from ancient times in India, as per Ayurvedic texts. Effort should be taken to keep the body clean internally, through proper detoxification methods as in occasional enema, purging, fasting, cleansing diet etc.

Holistic approach

Holistic treatments to delay ageing work at different levels. These include treatments from ayurvedic science, which has a special branch called panchakarma. If taken yearly, it is said to have proven effects on maintaining youthfulness, apart from the naturopathic treatments and yoga. Acupuncture and oriental healing techniques also contribute a lot in preventing ageing.

Whole body massages with medicated oils help to relieve stress, apart from maintaining your complexion and skin tone. It reduces the wrinkling of the skin and protects hair from greying, dandruff, and hair thinning. It improves the muscle tone and protects joint mobility. It also ensures good quality of sleep.

Homeopathy

Homeopathic remedies given constitutionally help to maintain health and thus prevent ageing.

Naturopathy

Naturopathic techniques like fasting and cleansing diets—when combined with hydrotherapic treatments including enemas and colon hydrotherapy—ensure proper internal cleansing. This should be done on a regular basis as per medical advice. Hydrotherapy, massages, fruit and vegetable packs, and mud baths help improve the skin and the internal organ function.

Acupuncture is widely sought after in present days, to overcome the most visible sign of ageing—the wrinkles. Acupuncture also helps in joint repair, to maintain posture, to improve sleep, to balance hormones, and for the general well-being of an individual. Oriental healing techniques like reflexology and acupressure help in deep relaxation of the nerves and stimulate the internal organs.

Ayurveda

Treatments such as Sirodhara, Pizhichil, Navarakizhi, and Patrapinda Swedam help in restoring youthfulness and vigour. Sirodhara has a positive effect on stress and strengthens the nervous system. It has an effect on the autonomic nervous system and also the pituitary system which controls the hormone secretions in the body. And as we all know, hormones play a great role in maintaining youthfulness.

Pizhichil, Navarakizhi, and Patrapinda Swedam have a deep acting effects on the changes with ageing happening in the cells and tissues. These treatments not only reverse the changes, but also prevent or delay it, if taken regularly. Ayurvedic Panchakarma treatments taken as per one's constitution and symptoms are most effective in delaying the ageing process too.

Capsule Gandha Tailam taken on a regular basis helps

restoring bone strength and preventing degenerative changes. Soubhagya Shunti Pakam, Satavari Gulam, and Balarishtam help in dealing with menopausal symptoms and restoring female health. Rasayana treatments can be done on a regular basis.

Yoga

Yoga has a holistic perspective and acts as a preventive and curative aid in the ageing process. It works at the physical, mental, and spiritual levels. It is the best practice to prevent reduction in height and altered posture, which generally happens as a result of ageing. Suryanamaskars and pranayama like Brahmari, Kapalabhati, and Nadi Shodhana help to prevent the ageing process.

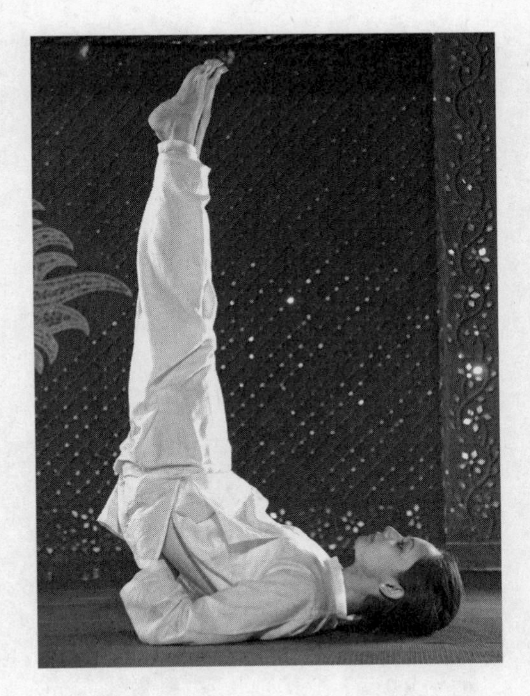

Vipareeta Karani Asana (both leg raising)

- Lie down face up, legs together, hands by the side of the body.
- Let the palms face the ground.
- Inhale and raise both the legs up, if possible to 90 degrees.
- Make sure the knees are not bent.
- If you feel a strain in the back, place the palms beneath the hips.
- Hold the posture with normal breathing.
- You start to feel the tightening of the abdominal muscles.
- With an exhalation, slowly bring the legs to the ground, without any jerks.
- Keep the legs apart, hands away from the body and relax.

Benefit

Here circulation is drawn towards the abdominal region, thus improving the digestion and toning the abdominal muscles

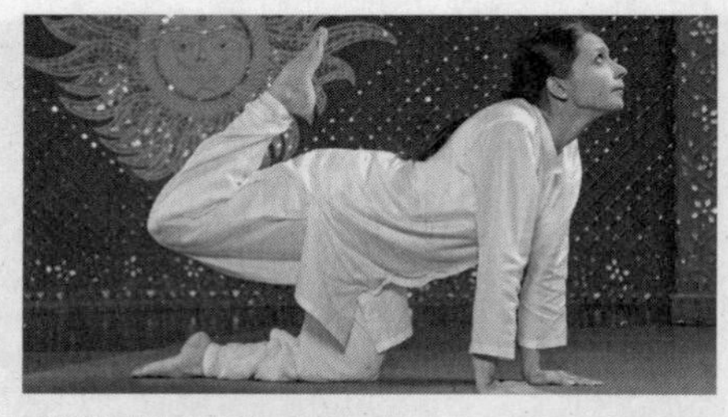

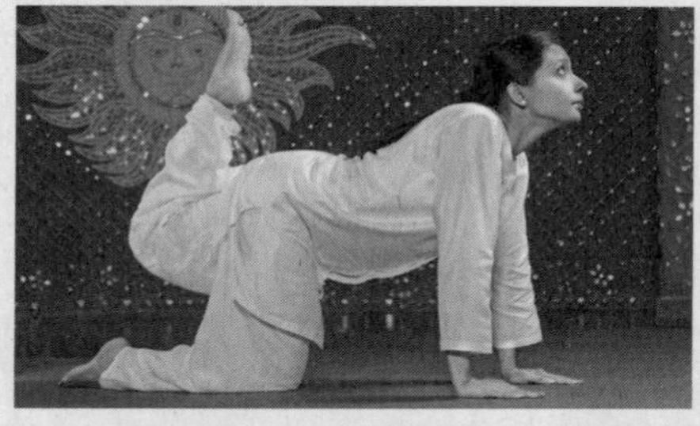

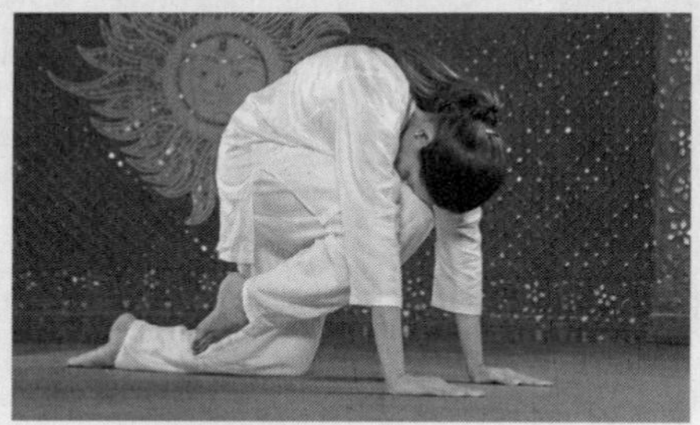

Vyagrasana

- Sit on all fours.
- Let the palms be placed a comfortable distance away in the front of the knees.
- Let the knees be placed apart.
- With an inhalation, push the spine in and lift the head up. Simultaneously lift one leg up, bend the knee such that the toes point to the crown of your head.
- When you exhale, lift up your spine and bend the head down, bring the knee from under the hip and touch the knee to the tip of the nose.
- Repeat this for few breaths with each leg.

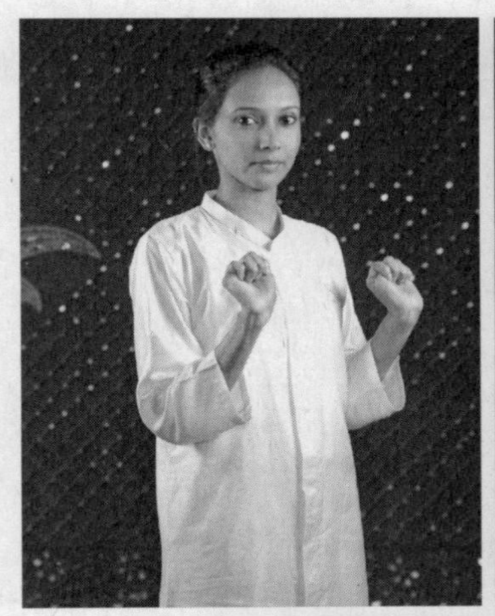

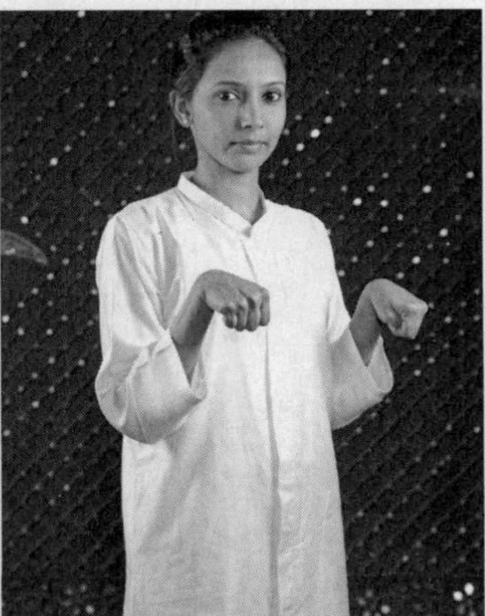

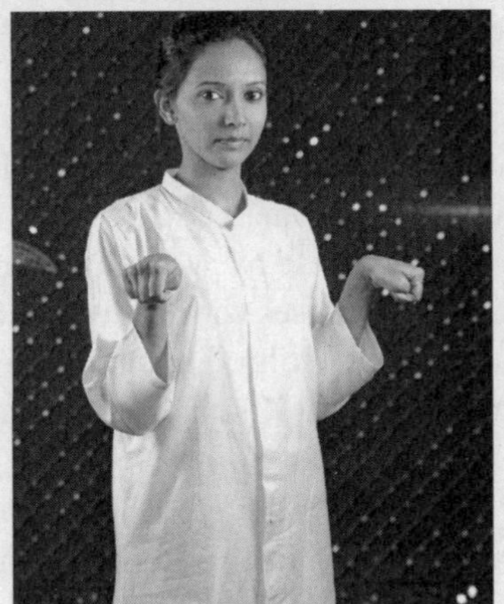

Wrist movements

1. Lock the elbows.
2. Make a fist of the hands
3. Move the hands up and down slowly, then to the sides and then do the rotation in both the directions. Let the movements be slow.

Conclusion

IT WAS MY DREAM TO WRITE A BOOK DEDICATED TO women's health since childhood when I would see my mother tirelessly run a humble homeopathic clinic in my native town. She was the only doctor in the forest-dominated Wayanad, Kerala. Very often, difficult cases that were almost dismissed as fatal by allopathic doctors were brought to her. I remember I would see patients walk into her clinic in the middle of the night and she would treat them with a smile on her face.

I learnt a great deal just by watching her. Even though I live on the SOUKYA premises with my wife Suja and our three kids, Anna, Mathew, and John, I make it a point to take time off to be with my mother in Kerala very often. She will always be my source of inspiration.

Over the years, I have realized how women's health is such an overlooked topic in this country. In today's world, women are juggling multiple roles—from primary caretakers to corporate managers, women are constantly working. And that takes a toll on their health, sooner or later.

When I established my holistic health centre in the late 90s, people ridiculed me. They said I was making a grave mistake by investing so much time and money in the centre. But I did not give in and stuck to my decision. I'm glad I did! I have now been practicing for over 25 years, and have a patient network from over 80 countries.

I have seen patients come to me after all else has failed. But I am no miracle worker. My team of doctors and I counsel each patient, integrating different systems of medicine like ayurveda, homeopathy, naturopathy, yoga therapy and supplemented by complementary therapies like acupuncture, hydrotherapy etc. We bring in allopathic consultants like cardiologists, neurologists, psychologists, and psychiatrists wherever the situation demands it.

Today I see so many doctors indulging in medical malpractices just to make a quick buck. But in the process, they also exploit the hapless patient, submitting him to irrelevant tests, and prescribing drugs that he doesn't even require in the first place!

But in homeopathy, ayurveda, and naturopathy, there are no side-effects. I will still caution you against self-appointed specialists in this field who prescribe medications with the promise of offering short-term relief.

I still firmly believe that there should be no barrier between different forms of medicine as long as the patient is cured of his illness. Remember, it's not important which form of medicine cures a patient; it is the treatment which matters.

Listen to your body; promote your health, nurture, and pamper it—for it is your most precious gift.

Acknowledgements

This book would not have been possible without the support of my family, especially my wife, Suja, who has been a huge support to my dream—SOUKYA. She has made me understand the deep and multifaceted role of a woman who is not just a wife, mother, and daughter but can also be a selfless caregiver, a pillar of strength and faith, a patient listener, and a caring attendant. My mother, Dr Annamma Mathai, who has been the inspiration and guide for me to understand women's health issues and the complexities of life. My daughter, Anna, who as a baby girl taught me the need for attention, as a teenager sensitivity and love and watching her transformation to womanhood which has given me the deepest understanding of a woman growing up. My sons, Mathew and John, in whom I revisited my childhood, and for their patience when I took time to write the book.

Lynn Franklin for encouraging me to write. Dr Sudha for her support. Dr Shubha for her support with the technical material and yoga pictures required for the book. Dr Ashwathi for her yoga pictures. Dr Sheeja for her compilation and inputs. Mary Faife for coordinating my time and schedule in order to make this book happen. And lastly, I would like to thank all my patients from around the world who have placed their trust and had faith in me for over 25 years, particularly the women who gave me the experience and insights into different issues that women face.

A Note on the Author

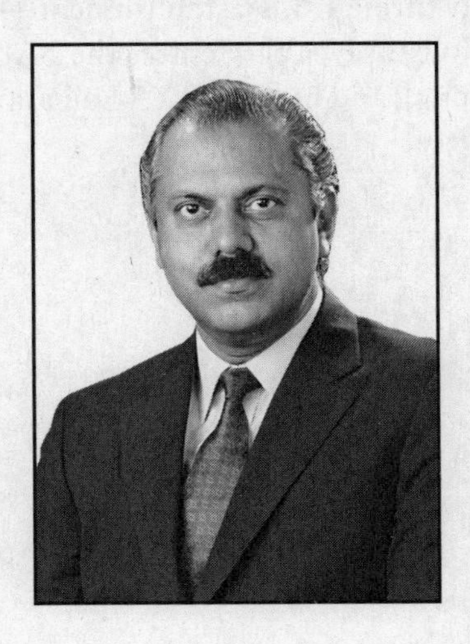

A second-generation homeopathic physician, Dr Issac Mathai is a world-renowned holistic health consultant treating patients from more than 80 countries over the last 25 years. He studied Chinese Pulse Diagnosis and Acupuncture at the WHO Institute, Nanjing, China, learnt Yoga and Transcendental Meditation, and has participated in the Mind-Body Medicine programme by the Harvard Medical School, USA. His rich experience started by interning with his mother, Dr Annamma Mathai and having worked at speciality clinics, including Europe's first and largest holistic health clinic, The 101 Clinic. He is a visiting consultant at holistic clinics in London, New York, and Washington DC. Having addressed several conferences worldwide on holistic health, he has been invited by the World Health Organization (WHO) into its committee for 'The Renewal of the Global Health Policy for the 21st century'. He has treated people ranging from Royalty of the UK, Middle East and India, Nobel Laureate Archbishop Desmond Tutu, famous singers, industrialists, CEOs, villagers, and tribals. His dream of offering holistic integrative medicine to all is fulfilled through his establishments—the SOUKYA International Holistic Health Centre, the SAHAYA Holistic Integrative Hospital, and his SOUKYA Foundation free clinics and charity centres.

A Note on SOUKYA

SOUKYA International Holistic Health Centre, the brainchild of Dr Mathai, is the first of its kind in the world where different systems of medicines like ayurveda, homeopathy, yoga, and naturopathy as well as complementary therapies are integrated with allopathy. Located on a 30-acre certified organic farm in Whitefield, on the outskirts of Bangalore, not only is SOUKYA India's first NABH accredited AYUSH Hospital for ayurveda, homeopathy, yoga, and naturopathy, it has also received several awards—the national award for the 'Best Wellness Centre' being the most prestigious one. The centre provides authentic, high quality treatment for all kinds of medical conditions as well as for wellness. It grows hundreds of species of medicinal plants for the in-house production of ayurvedic oils and medicines and for fresh use in treatments. Being a model for a holistic way of living, it also grows vegetables and fruits with its organic composting, vermiculture, utilizes solar for heating and power, wind for electricity, energy saving devices, bio-gas, rain water harvesting, drip irrigation, and utilizes natural light and ventilation.